STAYING CLEAN LIVING DIRTY

GAIL BRENNER NASTASIA

For my kids

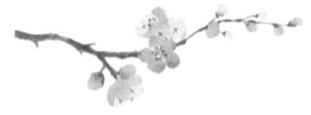

CONTENTS

2009

2010-2011

2012–2015

2002-2003

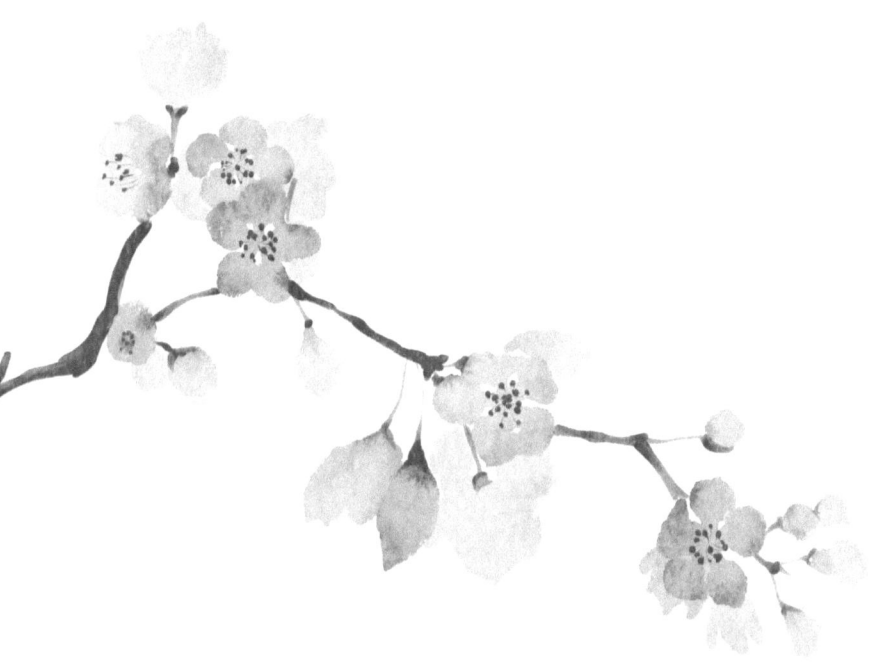

1

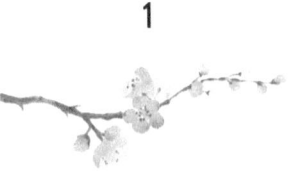

THE JIG IS UP

"I'm gonna be sick." Covering my mouth, I rush away from the harbor in a frantic search for privacy. There are people everywhere. Ronnie, my new husband of one month, is right behind me as I stumble toward the street. At the curb, I grab hold of a newly planted sapling and hurl until I'm empty.

When I finally right myself, I turn to Ronnie, who is holding out a napkin. He's good at showing up with what I need.

"Are you okay?"

"Yeah. It must be the pizza." I look away from him as I speak so he won't see the lie in my eyes. "And the heat," I add. But the truth is, it was Percocet that made me sick. For the second time in an hour, and the first time in my life, the pills refused to stay down. Ronnie seems to believe me. He doesn't know I relapsed more than a year ago. Nobody does. Everybody thinks I've been clean for a couple of years.

From just a few feet behind him, my son, Jack, looks on, his face full of concern. He's never seen me like this, and his expression reminds me of what mine must've looked like when I was ten, like him, and my mother would lie in her dark bedroom for hours with a cold facecloth draped across her forehead, complaining about a migraine. Even then, I knew it had something to do with the drugs. I wonder if Jack knows something too.

I put on a smile. "Let's get back over there. The fireworks are about to start."

THAT WAS YESTERDAY—the day the pills turned on me. We were in Gloucester, my hometown, for the Independence Day festivities—the July third Horribles Parade and fireworks—a tradition since I was a kid.

The day had begun with a rollercoaster of emotions. Gloucester visits always cause me anxiety, and as if that weren't enough to deal with, I'd resolved to push through it without getting high. After months of struggling to put down the drugs, it would've been my second day clean. It helped that I didn't have any narcotics in my possession. And getting them was no easy task.

All was well first thing in the morning. The bedroom was cool, and I was alone. Ronnie was already up and out of bed. I lounged, playing on my PalmPilot, until a little after nine when my need to use the bathroom forced me to get up.

Once in the hallway, away from the air conditioner's hum, I could hear Ronnie outside working in the yard. Otherwise, the house was quiet. Jack, my boy, was downstairs in the house's lower level. He shares the space with Alita, my oldest, who was spending the week with her father.

After making a cup of tea, I went to the living room to relax. With my steaming mug on the coffee table, I leaned back and lit a Newport. It was going to be a good day. I was sure of it.

But by ten-thirty, I felt a thin layer of sweat form along my upper lip, a clear sign of withdrawal. As I wiped it away, I smelled the fentanyl chemicals seeping from my skin. I'd gone over twenty-eight hours without putting any drugs in my system.

Half an hour later, well before lunchtime, my whole body ached. My lower back screamed and the contractions in my calf muscles felt like charley horses. Still, I was determined to power through it.

I made a second cup of tea, having no desire to eat, and sat at the kitchen table.

From my chair, I could see Ronnie outside. He was trimming the grass along the chain-link fence, shirtless, his Italian skin dark from the sun and his thick gold chain glistening. Even at forty-four, twelve years older than me, my husband looked good. It still felt strange to call him that—my husband. As I watched him, I thought about how much he loved me. And despite his being rough around the edges, as people would say, Ronnie was thoughtful. He certainly didn't deserve what I'd been doing behind his back.

I finished my tea, showered, and blow-dried my hair. All the while, my body screamed for a fix. Relief was all I could think about. I needed something to get me through.

At one-thirty, while Ronnie was in the shower, I closed the door to my office and called the doctor. When the receptionist answered, I tried on my best pain-riddled voice.

"I'm still having a lot of pain in my lower back," I told her. "I need a refill on the Percocet."

"Okay, I'll check with the doctor. He'll get back to you."

"Thank you," I said, wanting to say more to convince her the pain was real, and I wasn't just pill-seeking, but I left it at that. She could judge me all she wanted as long as the doctor wrote the script.

I nearly jumped when the phone rang twenty minutes later.

"Hello," I said in the weakest tone I could muster, slipping back into my role.

"Dr. Simmons called in a prescription for twenty-five Percocet."

Relief swept over me. It would be a good day after all. While Ronnie got ready to go, I had just enough time to pick up the prescription and swallow three of them. The Percs wouldn't give me the same hair-standing-on-end, tingly feeling as fentanyl, but they would stop the smell and the aches. Later, I'd take enough to get a buzz, but for now, I just wanted to feel better. I dumped the pills into my pocket so they wouldn't make noise rattling in a bottle and finished getting ready to go.

With my addiction taken care of, I was able to enjoy the ride. Ronnie looked content and relaxed as he drove with his left hand on the steering wheel, the other wrapped around mine on the console. Maybe it didn't really matter that he thought I was clean even though I wasn't. It certainly didn't seem to.

I turned to Jack in the back seat. He briefly looked up from his Pokemon cards and smiled, his blue eyes bright and filled with excitement. I took comfort in knowing he would experience the best parts of my childhood, even though he didn't have the kind of mother he deserved—the kind I wanted to be. Thankfully, at ten, he didn't know I wasn't as present with him as I seemed to be. And he was happy, for the time being, which was all that really mattered.

After Ronnie parked on one of Gloucester's side streets, the three of us walked along the parade route looking for a spot to watch the procession. I kept my gaze directed in front of me, away from the crowd. As always when in town, my hope was to avoid being recognized. It was the only real way to keep Ronnie from hearing anything about my past. Not that he ever asked about my history or seemed to care where I came from. He knew some things about me—that my mother had been an addict and that AIDS killed her—but he still didn't know about my Aunt Julie and the things I did for money when I was a teen. And I had no plans to tell him anything about those years. I'd made that mistake before.

I used to share all of it with the men in my life, like it was my duty to warn them about what they were getting themselves into. The last time I told a guy all the sordid details of my younger years, he held me and wiped away my tears.

"I can't believe your own aunt would do that to you and that men would use you like that. You were just a kid."

Six months later, after our relationship fell apart, he hurled my confidence in him back at me. "You're nothing but a whore," he said as he packed his things. I refused to hand anybody that weapon again.

Ronnie, Jack, and I found the perfect viewing place near where I'd watched the parade as a kid. Back then, Little Nana, my great-grandmother, would put on her glasses and button-down sweater and walk my sister Chrissy and me to the corner near her apartment to enjoy the production.

When I heard the wail of fire engines, I felt the same anticipation I'd had back then. And as I watched Jack dance to the steel band and bounce from one foot to the other, while waiting for the next burst of Tootsie Rolls and Smarties to fall from the sky, I remembered how normal it felt to be there when I was his age. For a couple of hours, my family was just like everybody else's.

And I loved watching my boy have fun. He needed this, especially now. It was hard to tell how he really felt about me getting married. He was too young to volunteer that kind of information, and I wasn't good at fishing for it.

Following the parade, we met up at my best friend Loni's place, where we could park, and walk the short distance to the boulevard for the fireworks show. Jack ran up the stairs ahead of us and disappeared through the door to her apartment. He was excited to see Loni and her five-year old son, AJ. Since the show wouldn't start till dark, in another hour, we had some time to hang out.

My first order of business was to take some time to be alone with my pills. Gratefully, Loni had invited a few other people to join us. With Ronnie and

Jack occupied, I wouldn't be missed. Not that it would take me long anyway. I slipped out of the living room and into the bathroom.

Standing in front of the small sink, I fished five of the round, white pills out of my pocket. As had become my ritual, I held them in my hand as though giving thanks to whatever had delivered me the relief that was about to come.

I watched myself in the mirror as I turned on the cold water and let two of the pills fall onto my tongue. *What the fuck is wrong with you?* The question popped into my head as it tended to do. I swallowed before responding with the usual answer, whispering it out loud: *What isn't?* Leaning forward, I scooped water into my mouth with my right hand. Then I did the same with the other three pills.

After drying my face and hands on a nearby towel, I looked at myself again. Although I wasn't feeling anything from the pills I'd taken earlier, my pupils were pinned, tiny dots just like my mother's had so often been. In fact, if my eyes were a paler blue, and my hair a lighter brown, I would look just like her.

Emerging from my bathroom solitude, I found everybody settled in the living room. Jack and AJ were playing on the floor. The others sat on mismatched furniture, talking and laughing. Loni prepared snacks in the kitchen. I sat next to Ronnie on the couch and waited. Soon, I'd be able to relax completely.

Ten minutes later, when Loni placed a thick wooden cutting board holding mountain bread pizza on the small coffee table, I felt the welcome return of my appetite. I grabbed a small plate and the biggest slice. As I gobbled the pizza, I watched Loni, her curly blonde hair bouncing as she moved in and out of the room with ease, carrying salsa and condiments, and offering soda. She was a force, I thought, who, unlike me, had no problem being herself.

I had just put my plate on the table and leaned back on the couch, when I felt a brief, sickly twinge in my stomach. I took a deep breath and waited for it to pass. For a moment, it seemed like I might be okay. Then a bigger wave hit. The nausea came on so quickly, I barely made it back to the bathroom in time to lift the seat before violent heaves wracked my body. It felt the same as when I'd vomit during my pregnancy with Alita, but I wasn't pregnant now. Something was wrong.

When it was over, I looked at the contents of my stomach floating in the bowl. Since it had been less than twenty minutes from when I took the pills,

I could spot their remnants amidst the pizza sauce. If I didn't have more in my pocket, I might have been tempted to fish them out. The thought of it made my stomach turn again, but I ignored it and flushed. I pulled five more Percocet from my pocket, downed them with a handful of water, and went back to the living room.

"Are you okay?" Ronnie asked.

"Yeah. Just a little queasy. I think I ate too fast."

He looked concerned when he put his hand on my knee. "I'm fine," I said. "Really."

"When are we going?" Jack asked. He was getting antsy.

"Let's go," Loni said.

Stepping outside felt like walking into a steam room. As soon as the warm air hit me, I felt like I was being suffocated. My stomach lurched again. I swallowed hard and pushed my soggy bangs away from my eyes before lighting a cigarette.

As much as I wanted to be part of the group, I hung back, letting Jack go ahead with Loni and the other half-dozen of them. Ronnie stayed with me.

By the time we made it to the harbor, I knew I'd be sick again. I leaned against the railing, breathing deeply, desperately trying to keep the pills down. It didn't work. That's when I got sick for the second and last time.

After, with the pills and food out of my system, I wasn't nauseous anymore. My body felt fine. But I was overcome with a heavy sense of dread. The pills had turned on me. While the fireworks lit up the sky, my fingers traced the outline of the twelve remaining painkillers in my jeans pocket. There were plenty left, enough to try again. But it wouldn't matter. My body would reject them. I knew it then, and I know it now—the jig is up.

2

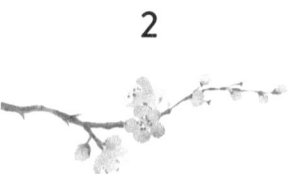

THEY SAID YES

I was clean when Ronnie and I met. By then, I was well aware of my pattern: I'd put down the drugs, find the cutest single guy in whatever church basement meeting I was attending regularly, and start a new relationship. This time, three months in, I caught sight of Ronnie.

"Hey, do you want to go out sometime?" I asked him one night after a few weeks of post-meeting meetups at the nearby Friendly's.

That Friday, he picked me up in his classic Monte Carlo, the T-top off, and we went on a harbor cruise. He stopped to kiss me in the parking lot before we got back into his car. Following a late-night dinner, we ended up at his place. Just like that, we were a couple, spending every night together.

I was hoping this relationship would keep me from messing up my life as I'd done so many times. Most recently, six months before meeting Ronnie, I'd been academically dismissed from law school. After all I'd gone through to get far enough to be accepted, I blew it.

I'd applied to law school before graduating with my bachelor's degree, despite fearing rejection because of my criminal record and past drug use. Those things made me the kind of person who needed a lawyer, not the kind who became a lawyer. I was also a high school dropout with a GED. But with over four years sober, and having worked with a lawyer friend I'd met in twelve-step meetings, I figured I'd give it a shot.

As far-fetched as it seemed for a welfare, food-stamp-receiving, single mother of two young children to succeed with such a lofty goal, I wanted it badly. My desire to help those like me, the people who'd been born into the bottom of the shit-pile, had become a central theme in my future-life fantasy. But what I secretly hoped for, what I really wanted, was for people to see me as a person of value. And Suffolk Law School had said yes. I was going to be a lawyer. It was my chance to show everybody that I wasn't a druggie loser.

But by the time the acceptance letter came in the mail, I was living in North Andover, a forty-five minute drive from Gloucester, feeling lonelier than ever. Although the move had felt necessary after my mother's death the previous October, now it seemed reckless. I didn't know anybody in the area.

That's when I met Rick, the brother of a friend. He was a few years older than me, divorced with two children. And he had a drinking problem. With over four years clean and sober, I wasn't at all attracted to him at first. But whenever we were in the same room, he made every effort to get close to me.

So when Rick stopped by my apartment one night for a visit, I invited him in. We sat on the couch and talked while Van Morrison played on the boom box.

"Come on, tootsie," he said. "Just give me a chance. You won't regret it."

"I don't know. I'll think about it."

When "Into the Mystic" began to play, Rick stood and held out his hand. "Let's dance."

"I'm not going to dance in my living room."

He held his pose. It was his determination that got me. I took his hand, and we danced. A few weeks later, we were spending every day together—him with his two kids and me with mine.

A month into our budding relationship, as we stood in his kitchen, Rick pulled an orange prescription pill bottle out of his jacket pocket. My stomach did a flip.

I moved closer. "What's that?"

"Percocet. I have a slipped disc in my back."

"Oh. Can I have one? I have a headache," I said, almost without thinking.

He handed me the pill as though it were an aspirin. In his defense, he didn't know how long I'd been clean or just how much pain that one pill would inevitably cause me. I didn't either. I convinced myself it would be okay. That I deserved to feel good. During the four and a half years I'd been without drugs, I'd lost so much, including my mother and Jack, the man I'd loved. Besides, it was just one tiny pill.

Just before the start of classes at Suffolk Law, less than a month after taking that first painkiller, I was taking them daily. Fentanyl found me a few months after that. At first, I did a pretty good job of pretending to hold it all together. Then, it all fell apart.

The academic probation warning came at the end of my first semester. It said something like this: if you don't get your act together, we'll throw you out. As much as the threat terrified me, since I'd yet to fail at college, I couldn't stop getting high. At the end of my third semester, I got the dismissal letter.

I appealed. There was no plan B. Without law school, I'd never be a lawyer, and without that, I had no purpose or hope for my future. It had been my one opportunity to prove I was worth something, even though I didn't believe it myself.

The appeals meeting at Suffolk happened on a weekday morning. I drove into Boston alone. While waiting, I gnawed at my nails, thinking about how I should've put on fake ones like I had at the start of school. Back then, they'd made me feel like less of an outsider, like I could pass for normal and people might not see the truth of what I was. But the bloody stumps at the tips of my fingers had always been a dead giveaway to the mess that lived inside me.

I'd taken a few Vicodin half an hour before my scheduled appointment. Facing a committee while in withdrawal was unfathomable. I was high as a kite by the time I heard my name.

There were two tables in the room, arranged in the shape of a "T." Each of the dozen chairs surrounding them held a body, except for the one sitting alone at the bottom of the letter. That one was clearly for me. Each of the faculty spoke: the dean, the associate dean, somebody from financial aid, my academic advisor, and all of my professors. All I heard was that I didn't measure up, that I wasn't enough, and that I was stupid to ever pretend I could belong there. My face was hot and itchy from the pills, and even if I had something left of my nails with which to scratch it, I wouldn't have let them see my hands.

"Do you have anything to add? Or do you have any questions?" somebody asked. They were all looking at me. I didn't have any questions. I hadn't even heard everything they'd said. And I was sure they'd already made up their minds.

"Yeah," I said. "Who makes these stupid rules anyway?"

The room was quiet. Even *I* couldn't believe what I'd said.

The dean broke the silence. "Okay. We'll inform you of our decision."

I stood so abruptly my chair nearly tipped backward, and I ran from the room before any of them had a chance to get out of their seats. I never told them about the pills, or later about my recovery. I'd like to think they would've given me another chance had I been honest with them. But I couldn't tell them the truth. It would confirm what they already believed about me: I didn't belong there. Of course, they were right. I was more convinced than ever that I didn't have a prestigious bone in my body.

The dismissal hit me hard. I had to figure out how to become a lawyer and prove I could be normal. Or pretend I could be. Either way, I had to be clean to make it happen, which is how I ended up back in meetings. Soon, I was able to string some drug-free days together. Days turned into weeks, and weeks became months. Then I met Ronnie.

Unlike when I'd been with Rick, my relationship with Ronnie helped me stay clean—at least for the first couple of weeks. His recovery and commitment to twelve-step meetings made it easy for me to do the right thing.

Then one afternoon, we stopped at Ronnie's house so he could let Harley, his rottweiler, outside. Ronnie's father, Tom, was there, working in the yard. "He likes to stay busy," Ronnie said before calling him inside for an introduction. The three of us chatted in the kitchen as Ronnie opened one of the cabinets, revealing ten or so orange pill bottles. My heartbeat quickened at the sight of the familiar containers standing erect like soldiers.

A few minutes later, when Ronnie and Tom went outside, I helped myself to a pill from one of the two bottles labeled "Extra Strength Vicodin." My plan had been to hold onto it for future pain, but I swallowed it before Ronnie came back inside.

At first, I took Ronnie's pills sparingly. Then, I started getting prescriptions from Dr. Simmons again, and I replaced what I'd taken. Ronnie rarely looked in the bottles. He only used painkillers for actual pain, since they hadn't been his drug of choice.

Within a couple of weeks, I was taking more of the pills than I could replace, so I started putting similar-looking vitamins in Ronnie's pill bottles.

I couldn't stop. When Ronnie took me to Aruba and proposed on our hotel's veranda, I wanted to tell him the truth. But I didn't. If I told him, I'd definitely have to do something about my problem. I reasoned that he wouldn't want to hear about it anyway; he'd have to break it off if I kept using, and he didn't want that any more than I did.

I said yes to Ronnie's marriage proposal and made it my goal to stop using before our wedding date of June 1, 2002. That gave me a year to defeat my addiction once and for all. Plenty of time to get clean and then married. Law school in between it all.

I could manage that. I was sure of it.

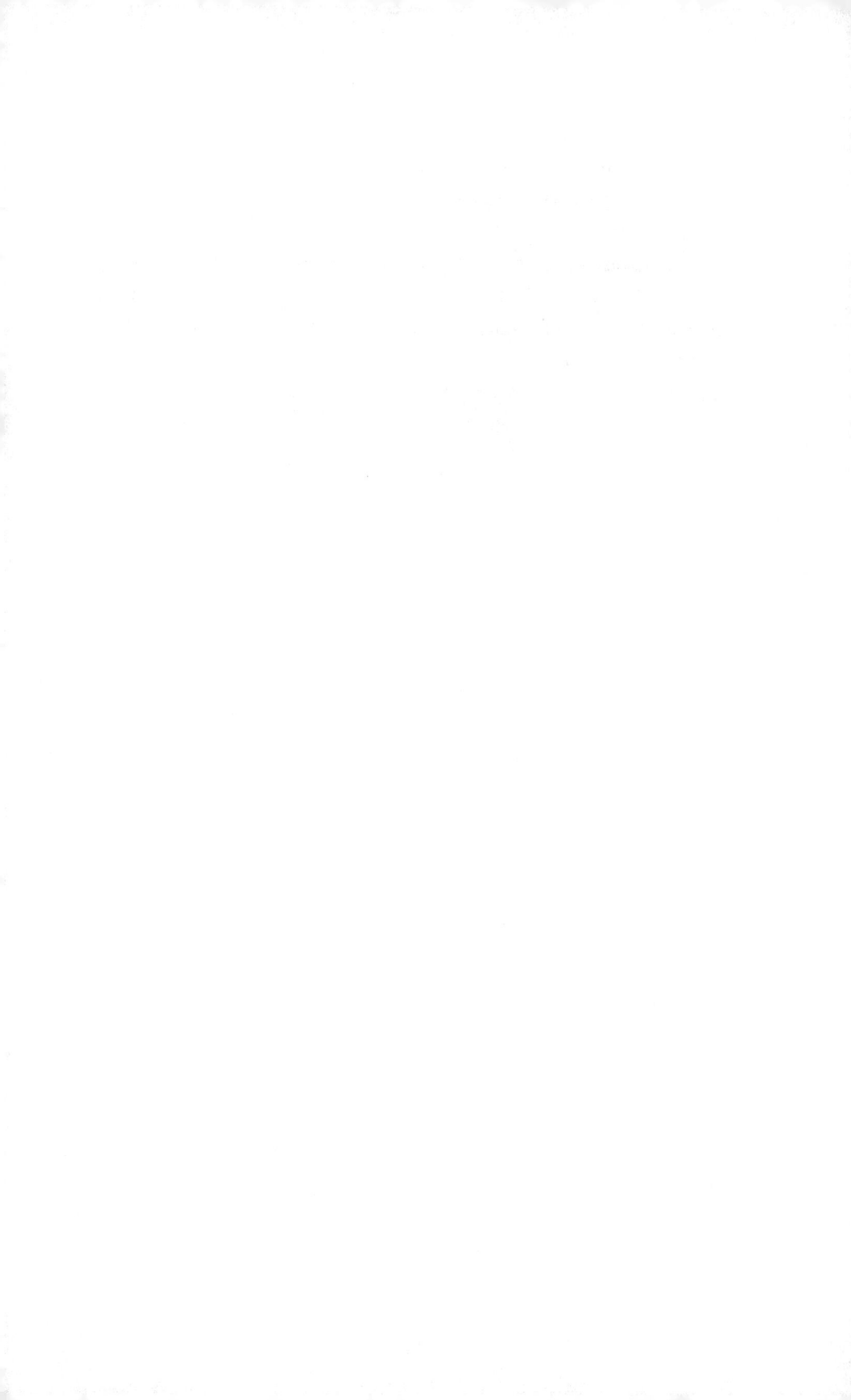

3

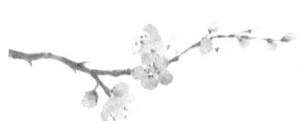

PAWN

A week after Ronnie asked me to marry him, I started planning the wedding. Having had more experience with funerals than weddings, I quickly became overwhelmed. There were so many choices to be made and things to think about.

Of course, Ronnie being religious, the actual ceremony would be in the Catholic church. Then there was the reception venue, music, dress, photographer, flowers, favors, guest list—oh, and the rings. So much I'd never even considered.

Growing up, I didn't think about getting married at all, never mind an actual wedding. While other girls my age fantasized about their white weddings, I was looking for a place to sleep. Then, as an adult with two kids, I figured if I ever did get married, the most I could hope for was an exchange of vows at City Hall. But Ronnie, having a big Italian family, wanted a big wedding. So a big wedding it was.

Before long, I was using more than ever. And, same as always, I got on the I'll-stop-tomorrow plan. With my legal prescriptions limited to just one doctor, there were times when I couldn't find any opiates. On those days, I'd have to settle for something else like Gabapentin or Xanax. With those kinds of drugs, I had little control over how high I'd get.

One Saturday afternoon, when the only thing I could find was Gabapentin, I took three before Ronnie and I went to tour a potential reception location. I felt clear as we trailed behind the event coordinator—a no-nonsense woman whose pleated pants and long sleeves suggested she took weddings very seriously—as she toured us through the hall. By the time she led us into her office, the pills had kicked in. The rest of the day was a blur.

The following afternoon, while sitting alone at the kitchen table wrapping lavender tulle around the heart-shaped candle wedding favors, I had a sudden spark of memory of Ronnie and me at the reception venue. While attempting to sit in a chair in front of the woman's desk, I swayed as my purse strap caught on the arm. When I pulled at it, both the chair and I nearly toppled over. I caught myself and sat hard on the seat.

At first, I remembered only snippets, like recalling a movie I'd seen long ago. Ronnie and I, sitting side-by-side in front of the desk, the woman across from us, both of them looking at me as though I were the opening act of a sideshow.

Then I remembered more. We were looking at packages and prices. I knew I was high and should keep my mouth shut, but I had my bride-to-be part to play.

"So, what are the hores de vores?" I asked, reading from the paper in my hands, sounding out the words and saying them exactly as they're spelled.

"I'm sorry?" the woman asked, her eyebrows coming together in confusion.

What doesn't she get? I wondered.

Then I saw her face change as it registered understanding. "Oh," she said. "Hors d'oeuvres." Of course, she pronounced it correctly.

Even though I was alone with the memory, I felt the heat of embarrassment in my cheeks. I wondered if Ronnie had noticed my strange behavior, and whether he realized I was getting high. What if he canceled the wedding? I'd been expecting him to confront me about using, and now I was certain of it.

AS EACH MILESTONE passed—my birthday, Halloween, Thanksgiving, and Christmas—I promised myself I'd be clean by the next one. I went to twelve-step meetings with and without Ronnie, and I kept my secret. When called on to share, I pretended to be sober. Once, I even told my story from the podium to nearly one hundred people because I couldn't refuse without tipping Ronnie off. I lied to them all.

One day in early January, five months before the wedding, I attempted to stop cold turkey. A late New Year's resolution, I told myself. It was as good a time as any. Two days in, my calf muscles clenched up like tight fists. I was exhausted but couldn't sleep. But that wasn't the worst of it. The physical withdrawal pain was nothing compared to the relentless loop of thoughts that spun around in my head. *You can't do this. You're just like your mother, and the drugs will kill you too.* I needed to make it stop.

Out of cash with another week before I could get a prescription refill, I considered all of my borrowing options. My boss, Peter, was first on the list. But I couldn't ask him. Being clean and sober himself, he'd surely know what I was up to. And I couldn't risk him telling Ronnie. None of my friends had any money.

You could sell something. I heard the words as clearly as if someone had spoken them aloud. That's exactly what my mother would do. It's what she had always done. When I was sixteen, Chrissy and I had pooled our part-time job money and had a ring made for our mother with each of our birthstones. We brought it to her on her birthday at the halfway house where she was living.

"I'll never take it off," she said as she slid it onto her finger, her eyes filled with tears. She showed the ring and bragged to the other women there, holding out her hand as though it were an engagement ring.

But a few months later, the ring was gone.

There was also the ColecoVision game console that my mother had gotten Chrissy and me for my thirteenth Christmas. We'd begged for the device, and, for the first time ever, we got what we asked for. Moving into our second-floor apartment from the camp we lived in over the summer, the gift felt like a solid way to celebrate our new home.

Although my mother never got around to getting a tree, the large wrapped package was there on Christmas morning, leaning up against an end table in the living room.

For the rest of Christmas break, I played the game as much as I was allowed, only stopping when forced out of the living room where the TV lived and my mother and her boyfriend slept. One afternoon, when I returned from school, my mother and the console were gone. She got home a few hours later.

"Where's the ColecoVision?"

"I brought it to be fixed," she said. She wouldn't look at me.

"What was wrong with it?"

"It wasn't working earlier, so I brought it to a guy."

"It was working fine last night."

"He said it was burnt out from being played too much, but that he can fix it."

We never saw the game console again.

I suddenly felt the weight of the gold bracelet dangling from my wrist. A gift from Ronnie. My mind drifted to the day he'd given it to me, his newly discovered generosity a welcome surprise. In the short time we'd known each other, I'd yet to see that side of him. That night, he had let himself into my apartment. We'd been seeing each other for a couple of months, and he'd been staying overnight. Of course, the kids didn't know that yet. After my last fiasco of a relationship, I was trying to be careful.

Ronnie wrapped his arms around my waist when I greeted him at the door. I took in the smell of his cologne; he always smelled so good. We moved to the couch, he sat beside me, and pulled a slender rectangular package from his coat pocket.

"Happy birthday," he said, handing it to me.

"Oh my God, I can't believe you remembered."

"Of course I remembered. Open it."

I felt like a kid on Christmas morning, although this was so much better than any Christmas I had ever had. I couldn't remember the last time somebody had given me a birthday present. Even as a kid, it was rare for me to receive anything, on my birthday or otherwise. I loved the way it felt to be thought of.

Slowly, I tore the paper away and found a white box underneath. Inside, there was a gold bracelet that sparkled in the lamplight as I lifted it from its bed of cotton. It was shiny and dainty, and I thought it might be the most beautiful piece of jewelry I had ever seen. I felt like I might cry. I wondered what he would think if I did—if he'd realize I wasn't accustomed to receiving gifts because I wasn't worthy. He couldn't know, at least as far as I was concerned, that what you saw wasn't always what you got.

"Do you like it?"

"I love it." I thanked him as I took the chain out of the box and held out my hand for him to help me with the clasp.

I felt lucky to have him. It made me think that maybe I could have a genuine relationship with somebody who truly wanted a life with me and my kids. Ronnie was exactly the kind of guy I needed—a clean and sober man who was living a good life.

No, I couldn't part with the bracelet. It was too important. And I knew what it felt like to have somebody pawn a gift you'd given them.

I suddenly remembered the Black & Decker drill I'd gotten Ronnie for Christmas. He was so good at gift-giving, and I wanted to make him as happy as he'd made me. But he was so hard to buy for—he had enough money to get anything he wanted, and that's what he did. And since there was nothing he needed, I tried to get creative. I hadn't seen him do much in the way of home improvement, but what guy doesn't like a drill?

After opening the gift on Christmas morning, he thanked me in the same way I used to thank my Aunt Sherry when I'd hold up whatever matching pajamas or socks she'd gotten my sister and me that year. Maybe he didn't hate it, but he certainly didn't love it. He put the unopened box in the lower kitchen cabinet with his other tools, near where he stored his pills.

Grateful that Ronnie was still at work and the kids were at school, I nearly skipped the short distance from the living room to the kitchen. There it was, right where Ronnie had left it. I gently removed the box from its resting place and fished the receipt out of my wallet. I'd hung onto it just in case Ronnie wanted to return the drill for something else. For that, I was grateful. I couldn't have gotten cash without it.

I put the box in a shopping bag, slipped on my shoes, and was just about to go out the door when the thought crossed my mind that what I was about to do was no different than what my mother had done. She'd taken something from me that I couldn't get back. A sense of permanence, the kind of stability that comes with knowing something or someone will be in the same place I left it.

The thought that came next was that this was different. I would replace the drill before he knew it was gone, just like I'd done with the pills. For a moment, I wondered whether my mother thought the same thing about the ring and the ColecoVision, but I pushed that thought right out of my head.

An hour later, I had thirty dollars in my pocket, enough for three pills to get me through to the next day. By the end of the week, the new, identical drill was in the cabinet, and Ronnie was none the wiser.

4

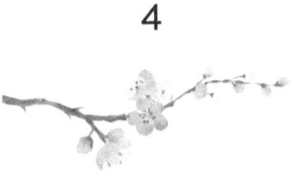

TOMORROW

The morning of my wedding, I woke early, alone in our king-sized bed. Ronnie had slept at a hotel, while I stayed at home. Knowing I wasn't as happy as I should've been, I was relieved to be by myself. There were still so many things I needed to work out before becoming a wife—like putting down the drugs. In the eight months before our engagement, and the year since, I hadn't been able to stop getting high.

The wedding day pills I'd managed to score were tucked in the pocket of one of my jackets hanging in the bedroom closet. Even though I was by myself, I'd hidden them out of habit. Needing them to do anything else is what got me out of bed.

As soon as my fingers touched the hard plastic container, I felt the familiar pangs of anticipation and disgust that accompanied my addiction. My body responded in kind; my stomach clenched and my throat tightened as though in defiance of what was coming.

I sat on the edge of the bed and counted out three of the big orange pills. I knew it wouldn't be nearly enough—the Darvocet was no match for the daily fentanyl I'd been using for months. Still, taking more than three was a risk I wasn't willing to take. I didn't know how my body would react to the pills; there was a good chance they'd make me sicker than I was already.

I didn't normally take pills so early in the day. Most days, I'd try to get through without them altogether. By ten or eleven, when my stomach and leg muscles would start to cramp, or I'd feel the other telltale flu-like signs of withdrawal, I'd try to coach myself. *You can do this. Just one minute at a time.*

When the cold sweats set in and the sour smell of my skin made me sick, I'd tell myself to make it through three days. *That's the worst of it. It'll be out of your system by day four.* But as my body began to ache from head to toe, screaming for relief, I'd give in. It was all I could think about.

I'll try again tomorrow, I'd say. *This is my last high.* It was the same thing every day, just like with cigarettes. And I meant it every single time. *Once this pill or patch is gone, I'm done for good. Tomorrow I'll stay clean.* But then tomorrow became today. And so on. Tomorrow never came.

Since I hadn't been able to stop before the wedding, the most I could hope for was that I wouldn't be sick. I downed the pills with a glass of water from the nightstand.

I cried during the ceremony and spent much of the reception in the bridal room swallowing pills to stave off the shakes and sweats.

I took the last three Darvocet in the hotel bathroom at Logan Airport, where we stayed on our first night as husband and wife. We were flying to the Dominican Republic the next day for our honeymoon. That would be my first day clean, I decided. Our honeymoon would mark the start of my new life as a married woman. And since I wouldn't have the opportunity to get drugs, it was the perfect plan.

Our first day in Punta Cana wasn't so bad. Aside from a few minor aches and pains, I felt okay. Early on the second morning of our honeymoon, a group of us crowded into a van for a full-day waterfall excursion halfway across the country. Despite sitting close enough to the air conditioning vent to give me goosebumps, I was sweating. The real withdrawal was starting. The trip that had sounded thrilling while planning at home in our air-conditioned kitchen now felt like torture. With the heat already an oppressive eighty degrees at seven in the morning, I would've given anything to go back to the room and curl up in bed.

The bus left us at a small airport where we boarded a puddle jumper for a short flight. As if the heat wasn't bad enough, the smell of fuel was so pungent it made my eyes water. That's when the dull throbbing behind my eyes kicked in. By the time we landed forty minutes later, I thought my skull would crack open like a walnut.

Trucks waited to take us to a clearing beside the road, where a group of horses stood with their owners. These would be our next mode of transportation, the owners our individual guides. We each chose our own horse. My pick was the one closest to me, a smaller, light brown female. The horseback journey was as harrowing as the plane ride. We traveled through the woods, across a stream, and along the edge of a cliff where all I could see were the tops of trees. I felt like I might vomit.

When we finally stopped in a clearing, the owners helped us off the horses before tying them to nearby posts. Ronnie and I followed the others to a weathered canvas-covered wooden platform that had been erected in the middle of nowhere. A jug of water and paper cups sat on its railing.

"The next part of this journey will be on foot," our tour guide said. Looking around at the other dozen tourists, I wondered if they felt as overwhelmed and exhausted as I did. They all seemed to be enjoying the day. I'd determined it was me. I knew I was the problem, and would've had fun, too, had I not been trapped in my own private hell. My body wasn't ready for something so physically demanding.

The trek was grueling. The guy wasn't kidding when he said it was steep. Much of the time, I had to use all my energy to keep from sliding down the path. Each time I had to stop to catch my breath, I promised Ronnie I'd quit smoking when we returned home.

"How far to the waterfall?" I asked the guide behind us.

"Fifty meters," he said. I didn't know exactly how much a meter was, but it sounded like a long way. And I'd have to do the same hike on the way back, except it would be uphill.

Relief swept over me when I heard the roar of rushing water. We were close. I picked up my pace, moving as fast as I could toward my salvation from the sticky heat. Just when it started to seem like we'd never get there, I saw the opening, and then the clear water before me. I stripped down to my bathing suit and stepped into the cold pool. For a second, the water felt so good I forgot I wasn't free.

Twelve hours had passed by the time the bus dropped us back off at the resort, and I couldn't wait to stand beneath the warm spray of the shower and wash away the sweat, dust, and chemicals from my skin. My bones and muscles screamed, and my head raced. And my experience told me that as bad as it was that day, the next would be even worse. Day three was always the most severe.

On the third day, it poured. Although grateful for an excuse to stay in bed, what I really wanted to do was join Ronnie in exploring the country. Having been outside the United States only one other time—when Ronnie took me to Aruba the year before—experiencing another country was what excited me most.

My addiction took that away too. I was far too sick to go anywhere. I needed to stay close to the bathroom. My mother's old boyfriend Walter would've said I was "dope-sick," like he'd said about my mother whenever she'd cover her bedroom window with a blanket and tell us all to go away. I'm not sure what he'd have called fentanyl-withdrawal sick, since he died long before the drug gained in popularity. But the sentiment is the same.

It was the worst feeling I'd ever felt. I thought about having a drink to take the edge off—a Kahlua sombrero or white Russian, the only mixed drinks I could recall from my teenaged years, the last time I drank. Alcohol was never my thing. I also considered dragging myself to a pharmacy in the hopes they'd have an over-the-counter something to ease the pain. My only other option was to search out a local with opiates for sale. But I didn't even know where to start. I didn't have a car, and I don't speak Spanish. The only thing I could do, the only thing that would bring me any relief, was sleep.

Just as I drifted off, demons and monsters came for me behind my eyelids. They ogled me with yellow eyes, their hairy hands and sharp claws reaching for me. My eyes popped open. I waited for my heartbeat and breathing to slow before trying again. As soon as my eyes closed, they returned. It didn't matter that I was wide awake. The creatures were as real to me as anything else, the faces of my addiction.

That was the worst of it. By day four, I was able to go to the beach and out to dinner with Ronnie. The physical detox was over.

I felt bulletproof when we got home on a Saturday early evening. With the drugs out of my system, and a much-needed distance from them, I was off to a great start.

On Monday, Ronnie went back to work. Alita and Jack went to school. I was already on summer break from law school, and since I was doing most of my paralegal work from home, I had some hours to fill. Determined to keep busy, I grabbed a handful of wedding cash and set out to purchase a new marital bedroom set. I'd never owned a new bed.

Halfway to the furniture store, the voice in my head started whispering to me. *I bet Donna has some patches.* I ignored it, but it persisted. *You have plenty of cash.* It was louder this time. The thought of it made my mouth water. *It's only been a little over a week. Start over again tomorrow.* It drowned out everything else. *Yes, tomorrow.* I made the call.

5

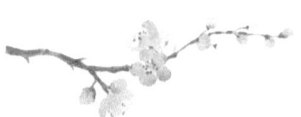

SICK AND TIRED

"I've been using," I say, looking down at my lap. Saying the words out loud makes my stomach turn. I'm sitting on Ronnie's side of the bed, the side closest to the door, and he's leaning against the dresser a couple feet away.

My decision to tell Ronnie the truth didn't come easy. Since getting sick at the fireworks last night, it's been the only thing on my mind. Over the last twelve hours, I've considered every possible option—leaving Ronnie, trying the pills again, secretly detoxing on my own, or finally being honest. Being honest made the most sense. I knew it was time to take action.

Leaving Ronnie hadn't really been a consideration at all. We've only been married for a month, and I want to stay married to him. I'm happy to be his wife. That had been the easiest option to eliminate.

The most painless choice would have been to take some of the pills I have left, and hope that, unlike the day before, they'd stay down. At the very least, they would've put an end to the body aches that began shortly after I woke up this morning. Maybe if I took only two instead of five. But I'm sick of feeling that way, and of lying. "I'm sick and tired of being sick and tired," as they say in Alcoholics Anonymous, and using every day feels like that movie *Groundhog Day*.

And detoxing on my own never works. I proved that most recently earlier this year during what was supposed to be a four-day spiritual retreat.

Ronnie went on the same retreat a few years back and was excited for me to have the same experience. Of course, he thought I was clean, which meant

I had to keep the truth to myself. I was nowhere near ready for anything spiritual, but I could only agree to go.

I decided to make the best of it. The long weekend away would be my detox. Not only would I get clean, but I'd get a jump on spiritual growth. It was a win-win.

I wrapped ten Percocet in cigarette cellophane and stuffed them in my pack. When Ronnie kissed me goodbye at the center, I felt strong, even though it would be our first time apart in the year we'd been together. The next morning, I dug out four pills, and the taper was underway. I'd take three on the second day, two on the third, and on the final day, I'd take the one remaining pill. That was the plan, anyway. They were all gone by day two. Spiritual wasn't at all how I felt as I sweated out the remaining two days.

So, my only real choice was to tell Ronnie the truth and put my detox in somebody else's hands. I've done it before.

At the time of my first hospital detox, I was fifteen. Back then, getting clean wasn't what motivated me to put myself into the locked ward; it was that I had nowhere else to go. I had been living with my mother and little brother, Philip, at one of her Gloucester apartments, when Philip tore off his fingernail on a door latch one night. My mother hadn't been home since the night before, and in a rare moment, it was just the two of us. I managed to get him to the hospital for stitches. When his treatment was done, I led him to the door. A nurse tried to stop us from leaving, saying that I was a minor and social services had been called, but I grabbed Philip's good hand, and we left anyway.

The next day, a social worker and policeman showed up at our door. "We know there was an incident with Philip last night and your mother wasn't home," the social worker said. "We have to place you both in foster care."

I sat at the kitchen table with my arms folded across my chest. "I'm not leaving. You'll have to carry me out." I'd already been to two foster homes; two too many, as far as I was concerned.

"Fine," she'd said. "You're old enough to take care of yourself." But Philip was another story. They packed a bag and took him away.

"How could you let them take him?" my mother asked when she finally came home later that day.

"What else was I supposed to do?" On the verge of tears, I retreated to the living room. I pulled half a joint from my cigarette pack and lit it. *Fuck her,* I thought. *She's the mother, not me.* Still, I couldn't help but think I was to blame. I should've done something like sat on the floor with my back against the door and my feet on the bottom step so the kidnappers couldn't get in.

"Gail," my mother said, snapping me back into the moment. "I'm sorry. It's not your fault, it's mine. I need to go back into detox."

"When?"

"As soon as I can get a bed," she said.

"What am I supposed to do?"

"You can stay here."

And then she was gone. A week later, the stragglers—people she'd let stay when they had nowhere else to go—had taken over. As hard as I tried to keep them from ruining the place, I lost control. I didn't belong there anymore.

Being January, it was too cold for me to sleep in my boyfriend's van, and although my great-grandmother, Little Nana, would gladly let me stay, I didn't belong there either. My Aunt Julie was still living there, and although I had told her I wasn't interested in making money with men anymore, the way I had been the year before, she wouldn't stop trying to entice me. Her presence made it impossible for me to be in the tiny apartment for more than an hour or two at a time.

One afternoon, while at Little Nana's watching General Hospital, I was struck with the idea of going into a detox myself. Why not? Maybe my mother was onto something. And, like her, I certainly needed it. I was getting high every day too. Well, as much as I could. Money was harder to come by now that I wasn't using my body to make it. And without money, drugs were difficult to get. Still, I managed. It helped that I'd take anything I could find. When it came to pills, I was like a dumpster.

The more I thought about it, the better the idea sounded. "Three hots and a cot," as my convict friends would say. I'd also get clean without feeling like crap. And maybe I did have something more to offer the world. Sounded like a perfect plan to me. All I had to do was call like I'd seen my mother do many times.

Less than ten minutes later, I was in the kitchen, dialing Gloucester's Addison Gilbert Hospital, which, along with those for the police and fire, was written on a sticker at the base of Little Nana's rotary telephone. I told the operator I needed a detox from pills, and after speaking with somebody on the detox unit, I called a taxi.

When I arrived, a woman at the information desk directed me to the second floor. There, a man wearing jeans and a button-down shirt asked me questions. I told him the truth.

"What kind of drugs are you using?"

"Whatever I can find," I said. "Valium, Xanax, Seconal, Quaaludes, coke, pot, percs."

"Do you drink?"

"Sometimes when I'm at a party or when I can't find anything else."

"When is the last time you used any drugs?"

"I took a Valium this morning."

He invited me to stay and handed me a clipboard. All I had to do was sign my name.

During my first hour as a patient, I bathed in the warm feeling of acceptance. I wandered from the smoking room to the milieu and back to the smoking room, introducing myself to my new friends. Then withdrawal started to kick in. I hadn't had anything since morning, and I was beginning to feel trapped. Halfway through the second hour, I was ready to go home.

But my signature meant a four-day commitment. Panic consumed me until a nurse handed me my first dose of methadone. The small cup of pink liquid made everything better.

That's when I started making lists. In a notebook, I created categories—school, home, health, money—and wrote what I needed to do under each. I'd been out of school for over a year, too far behind for regular high school, so I added: *find out how to get back into the alternative school.* The lists gave me a way to participate in my future and have some control over my life.

Four days later, when they still refused to let me go, I yelled and cried. Yes, I was a minor at fifteen, I told them, but I'd been mostly homeless for nearly two years. I was alone. None of it mattered. When the nurses and doctors looked at me, they saw a child. And social services, who was making decisions for me, wouldn't let me leave without a plan. I refused to go into another foster home.

On day seven, I finally convinced the social worker to let me go to Texas with my father. "He's sending an airline ticket to my grandmother's," I told her on the phone. In truth, I didn't even know how to reach him, but the lie got me out.

The day after my release from my first stay in detox, I sent away for a collection of pamphlets I'd seen at the hospital—the "I Should Be Happy...Why Do I Hurt" series. They were meant for adult children of alcoholics. Although I wasn't yet an adult, I wasn't really a child either. The lines were so blurry I couldn't tell where one ended and the other began. I was determined to stay clean and was hopeful they'd help fix what was broken in me.

They arrived too late. By the time the thick envelope landed on Little Nana's front porch, I was already high.

After a few more three-day spin-dry detoxes, I had my last real detox ten years ago. That time, I knew I needed more than a few days to dry out. I went to Adcare, my first and only twenty-eight day program. Long-term treatment had never worked for my mother, but I had to try. It felt like my only hope. And the decision wasn't one I made lightly; going anywhere for such a long time meant putting my kids in temporary foster care. It was the last thing I wanted to do given my history with social services, but there was nobody to care for them while I was away.

Two days before making a final plan, while still trying to avoid going that route, I went through my usual nightly ritual. I brushed my teeth and looked myself in the eye in the bathroom mirror: "You can stop getting high if you really want to." I said it out loud as if to show myself I really meant it. "You've done it before."

The next day, I got fifty milligrams of methadone from my dealer and drank half of it. My body needed the whole fifty, but my plan was to halve it every day. It was gone that night.

I decided to go cold turkey instead.

Next morning, my resolve was stronger than ever. I opened my eyes to a feeling of hopefulness for the day ahead. I sprang out of bed and nearly skipped into the kitchen to make oatmeal for Alita and get Jack's bottle ready. At four, Alita was old enough to pick her clothes for the day while I dressed her baby brother and packed his diaper bag. We were ready when the horn sounded, and we headed down the back stairs, Jack in my arms and Alita holding my hand. A family—the three of us against the world. I strapped them into their seats on the bus that would bring them home again after a full day at daycare.

I had big plans for the day myself. I'd almost failed out of the fashion merchandising program at Essex Agricultural and Technical College, but I could still turn things around if I worked hard enough. I was determined to get my grades up. All I had to do was read three chapters for my textiles class and write a five-page paper for literature, and I had the whole day to do it.

The first twinge of withdrawal came when I stepped onto the second floor landing at the top of the stairs. The cramp in my calf was brief, but I knew what that meant—the worst was yet to come. And I was right. It happened again when I crossed the kitchen threshold. As I passed through the kitchen, I looked at the sink full of dirty dishes, the pile of laundry beside it, and the washing machine. There was so much to do, yet I had no desire to do it. I walked past the mess and into the living room, where my textbooks sat in a neat pile on the coffee table. My drive to open them was gone, along with my will to do anything. I called Adcare and climbed into bed instead.

Adcare sent a car to collect me the next morning. Social services had come for Alita and Jack the night before, which gave me a whole night to think about what a shitty mother I'd become. But it was okay; I promised I wouldn't be away from them again. That was a promise I kept.

My first three days at rehab were spent in the detox unit, where they gave me meds to ease my withdrawal symptoms. After that, I was moved to the recovery unit where I made fast friends with my roommate. I made the rookie mistake of confiding in her that one of the staff had cashed the biweekly welfare check I'd gotten the day before leaving home. The next day, she and her detox-romance, Frankie, left the program with my two hundred and twenty-three dollars, all the money I'd have until my next check. I thought about leaving, too, but after giving up my kids to be there, I couldn't do it.

Back then, I was afraid to leave. The night before my discharge, our recovery unit met for our regular nightly group. We sat in a circle, the thirty of us looking uncomfortably at each other.

"For those who are leaving tomorrow," the group leader asked, "What are your plans? How will you stay clean and sober? Who wants to share first?"

My hands stayed in my lap. Nobody wanted to hear what I had to say. Life sucked for people like me, and nothing was going to change that.

A man seated across from me raised his hand and started to speak. "I can't wait to get back to my life. My wife can't either; she's been carrying the weight of our family for too long. I'm going to go to a meeting every day and get a sponsor. There's no way I'm coming back here again." Some people chuckled; others nodded.

The leader looked at me. "What about you, Gail? How do you plan to stay clean?"

I didn't know what to say. From where I sat, my future looked pretty bleak. And as much as I wanted to be back with my kids, I'd be going home to a dirty apartment with no money and a bunch of past due bills. "I'm going to go to meetings when I can and try not to get high."

"You don't seem as excited as the others," the woman said. "That concerns me."

"Yeah, well, I know what it's like out there in the real world," I pointed my chin toward the outside wall. "It's fine in here, where we're all safe, with everything we need. But what I know is that when I leave, I'll be alone again, back to doing everything on my own. It sucks, and there's nothing exciting about it."

"Amen," said one of the guys. This clearly wasn't his first attempt at getting clean, either. Some of the others let themselves nod in agreement, but there were a few scowls too. Those were the ones I was sure would be back. They were lying to themselves if they thought being back in the world clean and sober would be easy.

My honeymoon last month was just another failed attempt.

Now, here I am, telling my new husband the truth.

"Okay," Ronnie says as he sits beside me. "I knew something was up." He reaches over and puts his hand on my leg.

His small gesture of compassion breaks whatever has been holding me together. Covering my face with my hands, I let the tears come. "I've been trying to stop, but I can't. I need to go somewhere."

"Where?"

"I don't know," I say as I wipe my eyes. "I'll call Kim and see if she has any ideas." Kim, my sponsor of over a year, doesn't know I've been using either.

An hour later, Kim has found me a bed on a dual-diagnosis unit in Lynn. And while Ronnie is happy she found a bed so quickly, I'm afraid. I haven't been in a locked ward for a long time. But for the moment, at least, I'm willing to do whatever I have to in order to break free from active addiction. I hand Ronnie the rest of the pills before I pack my bag.

6

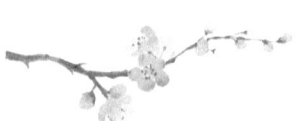

THE LAST DETOX

"**S**et your bag up here," says the same tall, sturdy woman who greeted me at the BayRidge Hospital when I arrived two hours ago. She points to an ancient-looking wooden table to my left. I do as she says and lift my small piece of luggage onto the table, the same luggage I carried onto the plane for my honeymoon last month.

Ronnie and Jack waited with me for a little while, but as soon as it became clear that my intake process wouldn't be quick, they left. I'm glad. There's no reason they should have to spend their Fourth of July at a hospital instead of watching fireworks. I hope that's what they're doing—having fun, enjoying the show.

The lady unzips the suitcase, flipping the top up against the wall. She removes each piece of clothing, shaking my undergarments and shirts, checking the pockets of my jeans, unrolling the socks and turning them inside out. The bag itself undergoes a similar, thorough search before she returns its contents.

"Put this under your tongue," she says as she places a plastic-covered thermometer in my mouth. She wraps a blood pressure cuff around my upper arm and pumps the rubber ball until the wrap squeezes tight. The pressure feels good. For a second, it makes me forget about what's coming.

Ripping the cuff away, she smiles. "Everything looks normal." I smile back, although we both know there's nothing normal about a thirty-one-year-old mother of two reporting for detox.

FIVE MINUTES LATER, a male staff member arrives to escort me to my room on the second floor. We walk along a corridor to the elevator where we ride in silence. I'm too tired to make small talk, and at the moment, I couldn't give two shits about the weather.

After going through a locked door, the man and I walk along another hallway; this one is lined with bedrooms. The place looks dated and worn, like it's been here since before I was born. And it smells just as old and musty. I'm guessing there are no open windows. But I have to be grateful, my goosebumps tell me there's air conditioning.

A few minutes later, my guide leaves me in a room on the right. I place my bag at the foot of the bed and sit. As I look around the room, I can't help but feel sorry for myself. It sucks that I'm here again—not in this particular brightly lit room with white walls and poor decor, but a virtual prisoner sharing a room with my cellmate. The only upside is that I'm alone for now. The other bed in this double room is taken, but empty at the moment. I'm not happy to be here. I don't feel relieved or saved. I feel like a failure, which is, I'm sure, exactly how my mother felt.

"How's it going?" The sound of a man's voice makes me jump.

"Fine," I say instinctively, before looking in his direction. It's not the same guy as earlier.

"There are snacks in the milieu if you want something."

"Thanks, but what I really want is a cigarette."

"Sorry. Last smoke break of the night was an hour ago. I can give you a patch."

"I'll take what I can get," I say with a chuckle. I don't want him to think I'm needy, but it's been a couple of hours and I'm already feeling irritable.

After he turns to leave, I lie down and stare at the ceiling. People are talking and laughing somewhere down the hall, and there's a television playing in the background. I can still hear an occasional firecracker in the distance. All I have to do is get through the next few days. Then I can go home and start the rest of my life.

IT'S BEEN THREE days since I arrived at BayRidge, and what I want most now is a shave. I haven't had access to a razor since I got here. My armpits are itchy and my leg stubble feels like sandpaper. That's not how I want my new husband to see me when he picks me up tomorrow.

Mr. Big, a floor technician aptly nicknamed for his size, is sitting behind the pony wall of the nurse's station. He's the same guy who doles out the comfort meds and takes us smokers outside every two hours. Unlike Addison Gilbert, there's no smoking room here. Of course, that was also seventeen years ago.

Since Mr. Big works so many hours, we've talked a lot and established a rapport. I'm sure he sees me exactly as I want to be seen, as a normal person who got messed up, and not as one of the crazies here in the dual-diagnosis ward.

"I need a razor," I say.

"Okay," he says, glancing up from his paperwork. "I'll let you know when somebody is available to come and watch you shave."

I laugh, sure he's joking. But he's already gone back to his writing.

"Seriously?"

"Seriously," he says, looking up again. "We can't let you have a razor without supervision."

"That's ridiculous." My voice is sharp, indignant, and my body is suddenly tense. I'm ready for a fight.

"Sorry," he says. "Those are the rules."

I can feel the heat in my face, and I know he can see it. I'm embarrassed and ashamed.

"I'm not suicidal." My voice cracks with the threat of tears. "If I wanted to kill myself, I wouldn't have checked myself into this place." I start to walk away, but turn back to him. "I'm a friggin' law student," I say as though that makes me sound more respectable than the low-bottom drug addict I feel like. But Mr. Big is unimpressed. He has no intention of bending the rules.

Fuck him, I think as I go to my room to wait for one of the female staff to come for the watch-me-shave-show. Thankfully, I only have to do this for one more day. I don't think I could handle any more than that. I'm ready to go home to my kids and to Ronnie. And I can't wait to get back to school.

I'm about to start my second year at the Massachusetts School of Law. I never did try to get back into Suffolk, although they might've let me continue had I told them about my addiction. Instead, I applied to MSL almost a year after the Suffolk dismissal. I was clean at the time, and in my application essay, I wrote honestly about my prior law school experience. MSL requested a meeting, and I agreed. I would've done just about anything to get my legal career back on track.

The meeting room setup at MSL was eerily similar to the appeal hearing room at Suffolk. I was seated at its head like Ward Cleaver at the dinner table. That was where the similarities ended. Sure, this was serious business, but unlike the Suffolk meeting, the faces of the men and women in this room were friendly. Of course, they did have an advantage that the others didn't: I'd been mostly honest with this group. My head and conscience were clear.

After some introductions, the dean began. "Obviously, we've all read your essay, so we know some things about your history. But we'd like to know more. I'll just let everybody ask whatever questions they have." He looked around the room.

One of the professors spoke up. "I just want to say that I think your honesty is admirable. It's brave of you to share all of this with us." Several of the others nodded.

"Thank you," I said, feeling strong.

"How long have you been drug-free now?" asked one of the men.

"Three months," I said, although it had really been a little less.

"That's not a very long time," a woman said. "Do you think you're ready for this? Law school is rigorous."

Of course, I knew exactly how difficult law school was after completing nearly three semesters at Suffolk; although I was high the whole time.

"Absolutely. I'm taking care of myself, and as long as I keep doing that, I'll be okay."

By the time the meeting was over, I already knew I'd be accepted.

Since I've been on summer break anyway, they don't know I relapsed again or that I'm in treatment. Classes will be starting back up next month, and I have every intention of getting it right this time. This year, I'm going to do things differently. I'll show up on time and sit up front.

I don't ever plan to come back here or to a place like it. I've had more than enough of graham crackers and decaffeinated tea to last me a lifetime. I'm going to stay sober. I should be with my family. And I need to be free. Maybe the timing of my being here wasn't a coincidence. After all, my sobriety date is Independence Day.

7

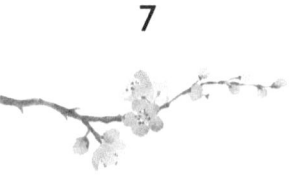

OUR FATHER

The aroma of coffee in the church basement makes me feel at home. I don't drink it, never have. I don't even really like the smell, but it comforts me. It reminds me of Christmas mornings when I was a kid and my family was still together; before heroin blew up our lives completely. Back then, my mother wouldn't let Chrissy, Philip, and me open our presents until she had at least a few sips of instant.

It's a Sunday night, and Ronnie and I are at our regular Alcoholics Anonymous meeting, the very hall where we first met. Since leaving BayRidge Hospital over a year ago, I've been going almost every day, which is probably why I'm still clean. Since Alita and Jack, at fifteen and twelve, are old enough to take care of themselves for the hour or two we're gone, this is our date night.

But that's about to change. I'm pregnant. After two miscarriages, one while I was still using, and another a few months into my recovery, I'm going to be a mother again. And this time I'm doing it the right way—married first and then baby. Ronnie's excited too. At forty-five, he didn't think he'd ever be a father. Everything is falling into place.

The setup of the meeting is cliché, with folding metal chairs arranged in a circle in the church's basement. So far, there are only a few people here, setting up and putting out snacks. We come early because Ronnie is the treasurer for the group, and he takes his role very seriously. Being here before the meeting begins also gives us a chance to socialize, since this is where all our friends are. And after seventeen years of attending twelve-step meetings, I'm more comfortable in this kind of room than anywhere else. Aside from a few of my remaining family members, Alcoholics Anonymous has been my longest relationship.

I STARTED GOING to AA meetings before my sixteenth birthday. I went to the first one with my newest foster mother; it was her idea. She'd been sober for two years and credited AA with helping her stay that way. Based on the things I'd told her about my history with drugs and drinking, we both agreed it couldn't hurt. But what I didn't tell Becky was that I already knew going to a meeting wouldn't help me. Although I'd never been, outside of my hospital detox a few months before, I'd learned from my mother that AA didn't really work.

Before Becky, when I was thirteen and fourteen, I'd move in with my mother from time to time—into whatever apartment she'd managed to get after her most recent detox or aftercare program.

She'd get me a bed or put a mattress on the floor, and I'd bring my trash bag full of clothes—what I'd been able to salvage after being evicted from the prior apartment.

At first, everything would seem perfect. When I came home from school, my mother would be home, cleaning to the music of Stevie Wonder or reading a book. Sometimes she'd tell me stories about her childhood and how she was learning to accept her past. Growing up was hard for her too. Her father walked away when my mother was young, leaving her with her alcoholic mother and no money.

She'd cook dinner before going out to an AA meeting. When she came home, her sparkling blue eyes looking directly into mine, she'd tell me about the "program" and how it was going to change her life. How it was going to change my life.

"It's helping me build the foundation I didn't get when I was a kid," she said. "And like a house, a family needs a solid foundation." I hung onto every word, hoping that this time she'd get it and finally stay off the heroin for good.

But after a month or two, she'd come home less often, and when she was home, we'd have more company. Instead of housing a gallon of milk, cheese, and vegetables, the fridge would contain only the post-relapse half-dozen eggs, maybe a stick of butter, some condiments, and a bottle of Pepsi. She'd never admit to using heroin, but when I handed a joint her way, my mother would take it.

Still, despite my fifteen-year-old feelings about meetings, I was happy to go anywhere with Becky, even if that meant suffering through an hour of listening to old people complain about their miserable lives. She and her family had already gained my trust.

So she led, and I followed her all the way into a huge, rectangular, brightly lit room. The sounds of people talking and laughing bounced off walls that were lined with folding metal chairs. Several tables formed a smaller rectangle in the center of the room. There was easily enough seating for a hundred, and my guess was that there were already half that many people in the room. I felt panic rise up in my chest. But as much as I wanted to tell Becky I'd wait in the car while making a beeline for the door, I didn't want her to be disappointed in me.

Becky saved our chairs with her purse and jacket, then led me to the cookies and pastries. I avoided eye contact, convinced everyone was wondering what I was doing there.

Once in my seat with a cup of hot tea and three Double Stuf Oreos, I reached for one of the nearby aluminum ashtrays and slid a Marlboro from Becky's pack. She'd already told me to help myself.

The room quieted as the speaker introduced himself. "My name is Ed, and I'm an alcoholic."

Everyone responded in concert: "Hi, Ed."

Ed continued from there, telling his story of woe. He'd drunk too much, and all was fine until he started to lose things like his wife, his house, and his dog. Bored, I took a drag from my second cigarette in fifteen minutes and tore my Styrofoam cup into small pieces. Nothing he said applied to me. I didn't have anything to lose, and I doubted I'd live to be as old as him; I guessed him to be thirty, at least.

"But it was the loneliness that got me here," I heard him say. My ears perked up. "I always felt different from other people, like I didn't belong. I could be in a room filled with a hundred people and still feel like I was by myself."

The hair on my arms stood on end. I knew exactly what he meant; I'd felt the same way most of my life. I thought maybe the meeting wasn't such a bad thing after all. I'd never liked to drink. Pills were my thing. But the substance didn't matter all that much since the feelings were the same. So I kept going.

Then they started talking about God, a topic which has always been touchy for me. It's been my biggest hang-up when it comes to twelve-step meetings.

It's not that I don't believe in God, because I do. At least, as far as it being something way beyond what I can explain. The farthest I get is that it created the universe and continues to play a part somehow. And from where I'm sitting, whether or not I believe in God, He or it couldn't give two shits about me. If He did, I wouldn't have grown up the way I did, living in the bowels of poverty and addiction, suffering through neglect and abuse despite being far too young to have done anything to deserve it. It makes no sense that I should now believe that the same entity that put me there is going to save me from myself. I'd say that's more a childhood fantasy than reality. And since my childhood didn't have room for fantasies, I'm certainly not going to entertain them as an adult.

Even though my logical mind wins out every time, I have tried to get on board with the faith-in-God idea. I've wanted so badly to truly fit here—to be all in. I want, more than anything, to feel loved and protected. Right from the beginning, I've asked people how to have faith.

At seventeen, I asked one of my sponsors: "How do I become faithful?"

"You have to pray for faith," she said.

"But how can I pray to something I don't believe cares about me?"

"Just try it. Get on your knees every morning for a month and see what happens."

I tried. Honestly, I did. Well, maybe not so honestly. I felt silly the few times I did it.

"I can't remember to do it," I said. "My intentions are good; but then I forget."

"Put your cigarettes under your bed. That way in the morning, you'll have to get on your knees to get them."

Again, I tried and failed. After a few days, I left my smokes on the nightstand where I could easily reach them.

Still, the meeting people have always told me to "just keep coming." So that's what I do.

I might not fully belong here, but I don't feel like I'm crashing somebody's party, either.

Then I met Ronnie, and I had an even bigger reason to try and find God. Ronnie is the kind of guy who never misses a Sunday service—unless he goes on Saturday. He gets on his knees and prays every morning and every night. All I can say is that if praying helps him to be less angry than he was before we met, I'm glad I didn't know him then.

Soon after we got together, I started going to church with him. I kneeled down at the appropriate times and sang along with the other churchgoers. We did our premarital counseling with the priest and were married in a Catholic church. But no matter how many Sundays I sit on the hard wooden pew, I still feel less like I belong there than I do in AA.

TONIGHT, THE MEETING starts promptly at eight. Chairperson Joe opens with the AA Preamble, before reading a passage from the *Daily Reflections* book. He then shares in his gruff voice: "I thank God every day for this unmerited gift. We are the chosen ones. Not everybody gets this." He then looks to his left, at Rachel, to signal it's her turn. It's a round-robin format.

Rachel, a middle-aged woman, identifies herself before sharing similar sentiments. "The first thing I did when I woke up this morning was hit my knees and ask God to keep me away from a drink, a drug, and a cigarette. That's the way I've been doing it every day for the last twelve years, and so far it seems to be working." Several people in the room nod in agreement.

A few people later, it's Shelly's turn. She's been struggling to stay sober for years. Apparently, she's been charged with drunk driving for the second time. "Now that I have to blow into this machine three times a day to stay out of jail, I'll have to stay sober. God is doing for me what I can't do for myself," she says.

This time, some people nod, while others laugh. I don't know what's so funny. Seems to me, it's the court, not God, doing for Shelly what she can't do for herself, and we should give credit where credit is due.

When it's my turn to share, I keep my thoughts about faith and God to myself. I don't agree with everything about these meetings, but I'm at ease in this room. For now, it's enough that these people understand me in ways most don't. They know what it's like to feel different—unworthy and unlovable. Maybe someday, like them, I'll come to believe in this God I hear so much about, and that He, or whatever it is, is looking after me, too.

The meeting ends promptly at 9:15, and we all fold and stack the chairs before forming a circle for the Lord's Prayer.

"Our Father…" I recite it along with the rest of them. If they are right, and He is listening, I certainly don't want Him to be mad at me.

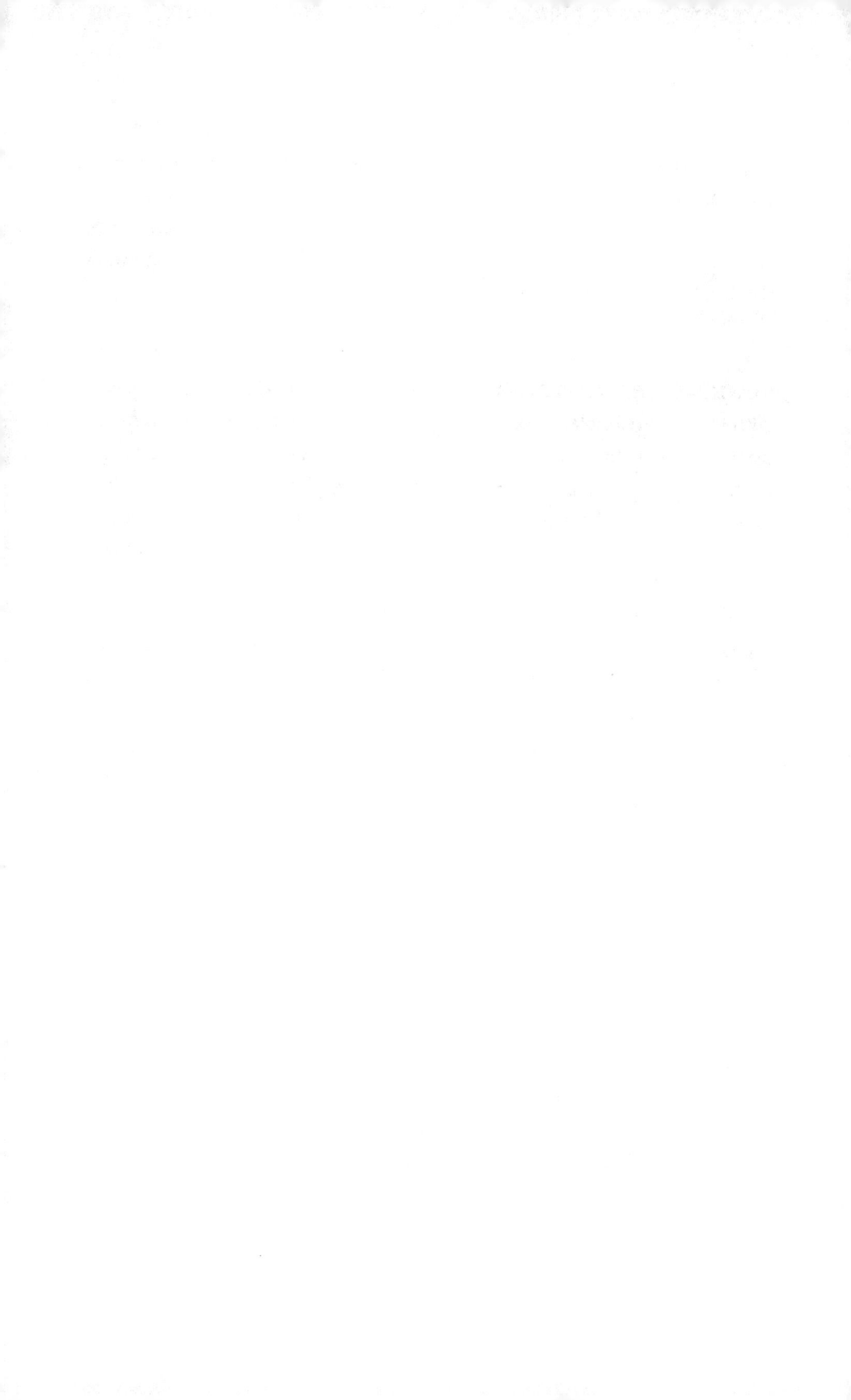

2004–2006

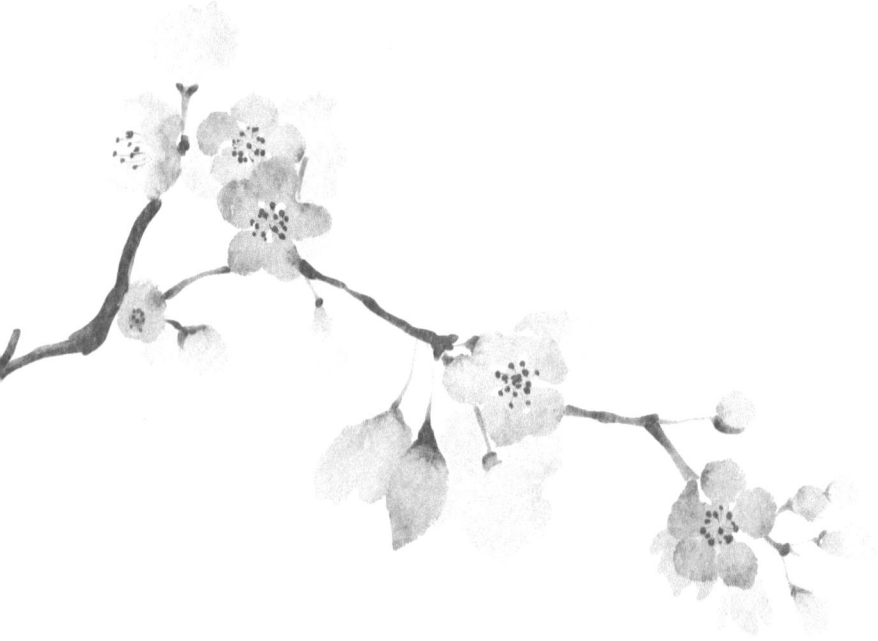

8

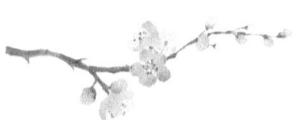

LICENSED

Today's the big day. It's my swearing-in ceremony. Ronnie and I are sitting in the back seat of my father-in-law's car. Tom is driving. As a former cop, he's the kind of guy who likes to be in control. Mary, Ronnie's mother, with her small, thin frame, sits beside him. She's as much a passenger in his life as she is in the car.

It was Ronnie's idea for us to ride in with his parents, and I reluctantly agreed. As much as I want them to like me, I still feel awkward around them. But they are my family now. And I want them to see that I'm not the loser they think I am. Yes, I was still on welfare as a single mother of two when Ronnie and I met, and I was still getting high for a while after we got together. I'm clean now, almost three years, and as of this afternoon—June 25, 2005—I'll be an attorney, licensed to practice law in the state of Massachusetts. Maybe they'll finally see me as somebody who's good enough for their son.

Gail Nastasia, Esquire. It still feels surreal. I've been working my way toward this day since I was twenty-seven years old, even longer if I count all the years of college before law school. It took so long I thought it might never happen. And with all the trouble I had between staying sober, the wedding, and then giving birth to Serena just two months before sitting for the February exam, it's nothing short of a miracle that I'm going to be sworn in today.

I'm sitting behind Tom, watching out the window, thinking about how I got here. I remember how grateful I was the night before the bar exam, when I checked into my room on the twelfth floor of Boston's Seaport Hotel. As soon as I got inside, I took off my sneakers, fluffed the pillows, laid down on the white, puffy comforter, and turned on the television. It had been months since I'd had any time to myself.

Ronnie brought Serena to see me later that night, and after they left, I studied for hours. I was determined to give the exam everything I had.

The next morning, I woke feeling ready. I sat with the other dozens of test-takers in an enormous room filled with long rows of tables, six deep. Electronics weren't allowed, and all other belongings, besides bottled water and something to write with, were placed along the wall in transparent bags.

Before we started the first day's multiple choice portion of the exam, I closed my eyes for my version of a prayer. *Mom, help me if you can.* Then, I opened the test and moved quickly through the questions. It felt so easy to me, that when I finished before half of the other test takers, I was sure I'd done something wrong.

On the second day of testing, the essay portion, I had less anxiety. I'm better at essays. Some might say it's because I'm a good bullshitter, but I know it's really a consequence of my love of words. I moved through the morning portion of the second day as easily as I had the first.

During lunch, a group of smokers were sitting outside. A girl with frizzy black hair and thick glasses was the first to break the silence among us.

"What did you say for the second question?" she asked the group.

"Foreclosures?" a guy asked.

"Yeah, how many elements?"

The guy stayed quiet.

"Four," I said. "I'm pretty sure."

"What about simultaneous death?" Frizzy Hair asked.

The guy took a drag of his cigarette and flicked it at the building. "I don't know," he said, before he turned and walked away.

I shrugged when she looked at me. I knew better than to go down the road of second-guessing myself, especially when we had a lot more testing to go.

When I got back in my seat for part two, I couldn't stop thinking about that girl. *Why didn't you just answer her?* Concentrate. *She was obviously stressed out.* Subject matter jurisdiction. Yes, the court has it. *You could've answered her. You knew the answer.* What about diversity jurisdiction? *Maybe. Stop. Focus.*

My head went back and forth for the rest of the exam. The only way I could stop myself from thinking about the girl was by shifting my focus to

Ronnie, and how he was doing with caring for Serena on his own. That made me anxious too.

By the time I turned in my last blue book, I was sure I had failed.

The two-month wait for the results was excruciating. At first, I imagined the worst: raising my hand at my favorite AA meeting to announce I'd failed and wouldn't be a lawyer after all. It felt terrible. So I tried the opposite. I visualized myself announcing I'd passed. I repeated it daily. By the time I saw my name on the passing list, it felt like it belonged there.

"My father's talking to you," Ronnie says, his voice nudging me back into the car with him and his parents. I turn my gaze away from the window to the rearview mirror. Tom's eyes briefly meet mine before he turns them back to the road.

"What do you plan to do after today?" he asks, apparently for the second time.

"I'm going to stick with bankruptcies," I say. Tom's been trying to convince me to do criminal work. He used to be a police prosecutor, and having been retired for well over a decade, he misses being in the courtroom. I have no desire to get involved with criminal law. Except to help out my brother. There's a warrant for Philip's arrest out of Gloucester, and he's asked me to represent him. He's been waiting for me to become licensed.

But I don't tell Tom that. He knows little about my family or my history, aside from having met my two siblings, Chrissy and Philip, and my father at the wedding. And as far as I'm concerned, the less Ronnie's parents know about any of my past, the better. It's dead and buried, and that's where it should stay.

"You should practice criminal law," he says again. I knew that was coming.

"No way. I can't even imagine doing a trial." Despite all the work I've done to become a lawyer, I still don't know if I have what it takes. I've always seen myself more as somebody who needs representation than as the one doing the representing.

At least, I used to.

9

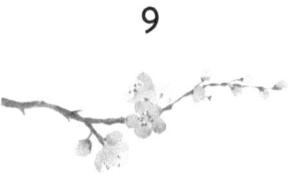

PUNKED

Acouple days after being sworn into the bar, I pull my Jeep into the only empty parking space in front of the Gloucester District Court building.

"That's a good sign," I say to Philip.

"I hope so," he replies as he puts his wallet in the glove compartment for safekeeping, in case he doesn't come back out with me. Even though he's a man now, over six feet tall and stocky, with thinning hair, I still see my little brother—the skinny, freckle-faced, five-year-old redhead. And I can tell he's worried. He has that same look on his face he had when Walter, our mother's boyfriend, found food in his toy box. It was the supper he'd been banished to his room to finish. Walter didn't make him eat it; instead, he gave him a spanking.

"I won't do it again," I heard Philip cry from the next room. I wished I could do something, like rush in and jump on Walter's back or call the police, but I knew my place. Being just six years older, all I could do was wait right there on my bed, biting my fingernails until it was over.

I wonder if he saw me as having more power than he had; which is, after all, how I saw people who were older than me.

Even today, Philip's anger is quiet but palpable. Maybe he resents me for not taking care of him when, after we were split up, heroin kept my mother away from us, or because he, too, was forced to bounce from one foster home to another while she was getting treatment.

In the years since addiction took my mother's life, we've had to work hard to stay close after spending so much of our lives apart.

Maybe he's bitter about the times I did try to take care of him—when I was a new mother at seventeen and didn't even know how to take care of myself. Despite knowing I was never in a position to help him any more than I was able to help myself, I feel the heavy weight of guilt that I couldn't shield him from his life experiences.

And now, I can't do more to console him. We're not affectionate. But I'm here, and the best I can do is try to keep him out of jail.

"I'm gonna smoke a butt," he says without looking at me.

"It'll be okay," I say before the door closes behind him, hoping I sound more confident than I feel.

Finally alone, I take a deep breath, trying to calm my nerves. I'm as anxious as my brother. Maybe even more. I wish I hadn't promised I'd represent him, but it's way too late to change my mind. This will be my first time standing before a judge where I'm not the one in trouble, and I was only sworn in two days ago.

As I watch Philip walk toward the building's entrance, I can't help but think about what could be waiting for me in that courtroom. My hometown has always given me so much angst—I still worry I'll run into somebody I don't want to see. I envy those who look forward to an accidental encounter with an old friend. Then I wonder, who would even recognize me from those years I wish to forget? I was just a teenager, getting money from men old enough to be my grandfather, in exchange for my doing things to please them. They were at fault, I remind myself. I was a child. I'm not even the same person as the twenty-five year old who ran away from this place—*Fish City*—close to ten years ago. Now I'm a married professional with a new baby girl; child number three.

I take one more deep breath and blow it out before opening my door to the warm, salty air. As I step out onto the pavement, I gratefully note there's no hint of the odor of low tide. It's going to be a perfect early summer day. If only I could get back in the driver's seat and cruise around the back shore with the windows down like I used to when I needed to unwind. But I made a promise.

I close the door and take in the mammoth red brick building before me. It is exactly as it was when I was a child.

As I move along the sidewalk to the entrance, I feel like I'm tracing the old footsteps of my past, walking in the shoes I wore when I didn't know my own strength. I pull my shoulders back and lift my chin. I'm a woman now, and I can do this.

The front entrance is covered. I walk down the ramp that hugs the side of the building, to a sunken plaza below street-level. The entire area is made up of the same red brick as the building. Aside from the gray cement patchwork on some of the bricks, it looks the same as the last time I was here.

As I make my way down the ramp, the sun moves further away. The entryway is as dark and dreary as ever.

Philip is standing to the right of the door, presumably on cigarette number two.

"Ready?" I ask as I reach for the large handle on the left side of the tall, black, double doors.

"I'll be there in a minute," he says.

I don't push.

Once inside, I take in my surroundings. I'm transported back to 1983. To my left is the police department counter, familiar and unchanged except for the addition of protective plexiglass. I also know what it's like to be behind the counter and to pass by the room where the officers watch live feed of the lower level cells. That's where they watched me after I was processed during each drug possession or shoplifting arrest, before I was brought downstairs to await my mother or Walter and their wrath.

Somewhere behind the counter is also where my mother and I met with the detectives who questioned me, a thirteen year old, swollen with poison ivy—about the men, the money, and my involvement in what they referred to as a "prostitution ring"—with no Miranda warning and no attorney.

"Assholes," I whisper under my breath, wishing I could go back and say it to their faces.

I scan the rest of the large vestibule. The bathrooms are to the right of the police, and directly in front of me are a set of winding stairs that lead to the courtrooms. A court officer stands at the bottom, next to a metal detector. He motions for me to go through as he's done for the others who've gone up before me, not knowing I've been an official lawyer for all of two days. I pull out my identification and temporary bar card and hand them to him. He smiles.

"You're all set."

I feel like I've just gotten one over on the guy as I put my credentials away. My apparent elevation in status feels like the best kind of high. I saunter to the stairs, my heels clicking on the tile floor, and make my way to the next level.

On the landing halfway up, I look through the dirty window and catch a glimpse of the harbor. I'm transported again, this time to an apartment not far from here, where the man who arranged meetings between fishermen and young girls like me stood in his second-floor window, watching for boats as they arrived in this very same harbor. The memory, like a needle piercing a balloon, deflates me.

The second floor, like the first, hasn't changed a bit, but it looks smaller to me, as things do as we get older. It might also be that I don't feel so alone and powerless anymore. Before today, I'd only ever been here as a defendant or as a child who wasn't being cared for.

To my left, at the top of the stairs, is the adult courtroom that was off limits to me as a child. Back then, while passing the room on my way to the juvenile session, I'd look inside through the open door and marvel at the excitement. The stadium seating was almost always filled, and the judge sat elevated in the center of everything. It was nothing like the juvenile courtroom down the hall, a small room dominated by an oval conference table where the judge sat at my level, just a few chairs away from me.

This morning, when I enter the courtroom, I walk directly to the clerk, a middle-aged man wearing a button-down shirt. He's seated in front of where the judge will be.

"Hi," I say. "Can you tell me where I can find a notice of appearance?" That is about the extent of what I know I'm supposed to do.

"On whose behalf are you here?" he asks while handing me the form.

"Philip Brenner." I feel a pang of guilt that I'm grateful for marriage having changed my last name. I'm able to remain incognito. "We're here to remove a warrant."

"Okay. Did he check in with probation?"

"No," I say. I can feel my insides shaking.

"He needs to do that. There's no judge today, not on Mondays. If the prosecutor asks for bail, I'll be making the decision."

I smile and thank him. I just need to sit and put my things down. It hadn't occurred to me that there might be a question of bail, since Philip's turning himself in.

I turn away to look for an empty chair. This is new to me too. I'm able to sit in the pen, the area meant for attorneys that is surrounded by a barrier I've never been allowed to cross.

Finding an empty chair, I sit as though I've done this a hundred times before. I'm sweating by the time I put my bag down.

I've just reached for the nearly empty file bearing my brother's name when I hear a man's voice. "What are *you* doing here?" he asks, sounding suspicious.

My head instinctively snaps up to face the much older man, who is standing before me. He's as pudgy as ever, and still sporting the same comb-over as when I'd last seen him. I recognize him right away.

"Holy shit," I say, "Mr. Dunsky." It's my old court-appointed lawyer. He represented me many times when I was arrested as a teenager. He'd also been my attorney when the court deemed me a child in need of services for truancy, when my mother was accused of neglect, and when I asked the court to emancipate me. "I'm working," I say.

"You work here?" he asks, his hands in front of him, palms up, looking around as though he's being punked.

"Yes," I say, smiling, sitting taller in my chair. "I'm a lawyer now."

"Really?" He pauses. "You passed the bar and everything?"

"Yes," I reply again. "Don't sound so surprised. Although I do remember you telling me that I could just quit school when I turned sixteen." I mean it as a dig, but I don't think he takes it that way.

"Well, congratulations. I'm impressed."

"Thanks," I say, feeling a welcome wave of pride.

Before Dunsky has a chance to say more, Philip walks into the courtroom.

"You need to go to probation," I say, facing him and the audience.

"Oh my God," I hear a woman say from a row close to the back wall. "Is that Gail?" I hold my breath and search for the source of her voice. I'm not sure I want to know who it's coming from.

That's when I see the familiar face of an old Gloucester acquaintance. Teresa walks toward me.

I stand to greet her since she's not able to come to me.

"Hey, what's going on?" I ask, wishing to avoid a lengthy conversation.

I have work to do, and it's clear that whatever has brought her to court this morning can't be good. Her eye makeup is smudged, her dyed-blonde hair is unbrushed, and her clothes are wrinkled. It isn't like her to look so undone.

She averts her eyes when she tells me she was arrested for drunk driving the night before.

"That sucks," I say. I think about offering to help, but I don't. It's all too much.

My head is reeling when I finally sit down, but I don't have time to think about it. I fill out the appearance form and go back to the clerk. As I hand it to him, he directs me to the prosecutor, who is seated at a table just a few feet away.

"Hi, I'm Gail Nastasia," I say, extending my hand. He shakes it and introduces himself. He listens while I explain why I'm here.

"I'm going to have to ask for some kind of bail," he says.

"Why?" I ask, trying not to sound as panicked as I feel.

"He's been in default for a long time, and these are serious charges. I'll ask for fifty dollars cash. I probably won't get it, but I have to ask."

I wish I could convince him otherwise, but I know he's right. After all, Philip was supposed to show up for court three years ago.

On my way back to my seat, I think about all the reasons I'll argue against bail. Philip is trying to get his life back on track since heroin claimed him just like it did my mother. He's been through so much and deserves a chance to sort this out. Yes, he's charged with assault and battery, but he was acting in self-defense—though I remind myself that's not why we're here today. We're only here to clear the warrant. If he does set bail at fifty dollars, I can pay it. I won't let my brother go to jail.

A few minutes later, Philip and I hurry to the microphone when his name is called. The prosecutor asks for the bail and gives reasons for his request. My insides tremble as I wait for my turn to speak. I wonder if I'll remember anything I had planned to say.

But once I start talking, I feel a shift inside me. Something strong and brave takes over, and I completely forget about being nervous. "It's obvious that Mr. Brenner wants to turn his life around. He came in here on his own, willingly, despite knowing he could go to jail. It would send a terrible message if you were to take him into custody when he's trying to do the right thing."

I hear Philip exhale when the clerk agrees to let him go with his promise to return on the next court date. I can't hold back my smile. After all these years, I was able to offer my little brother a small amount of protection. He needed me, and I was here. Not only that, it also seems like I might be okay at this job. Maybe becoming a trial lawyer isn't out of the question.

10

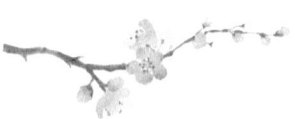

DEFENSE

In March of 2006, my first day of bar advocate training, I follow Andrea, an experienced lawyer who's spent years defending people accused of crimes. Even though I've been licensed for over a year, bar advocate work requires its own specialized instruction. Today, I'm here only to observe and learn.

As I watch Andrea in action, I wonder for the hundredth time if I'm cut out for this work. But after going to court with Philip and my father-in-law's persistent comments about criminal defense work, I finally gave it some serious thought. It was Tom who told me about the organization that helps people who can't afford lawyers. It reminded me of all the people from my past that I couldn't help. I applied at the end of summer. Everything moved fast after that: I had an interview, got the job on the spot, completed a week-long classroom training, and now I'm doing the in-court training.

Andrea first shows me around the courthouse, an old, small building with just two courtrooms. The main courtroom is dark and huge, with enough seating for at least sixty people. The small one, where they hold jury trials, is hardly big enough to keep the jury separate from the person on trial.

She shows me the clerk's office and the basement lockup that's accessible from the courtroom. Then she introduces me to the assistant district attorney, the probation officers, and, before the session breaks, she introduces me to the judge. As he tries to make small talk, I bite the inside of my cheek. I can't think of a single smart thing to say, and all I want is for the introduction to end so I can sit back down.

I'm so anxious. I thought I'd be more confident now that I've had some practical training, but that couldn't be further from the truth. Since being sworn in, aside from going to court with Philip, I've done some bankruptcy work, but nothing involving an actual judge. Being a defense attorney sounded much better in theory.

After lunch, I'm sitting on a bench in the courtroom when the judge addresses me. "Attorney Nastasia, would you be willing to accept an appointment?" he asks. I look around the room for Andrea, but she's not here. She must be in the other session. I want to tell him I'm not ready, but I'm the only attorney in the room who takes court-appointed cases, and I don't want to upset him.

"Um, of course," I say as I stand and make my way to the table where all the other lawyers have stood when their cases were called.

"I'm asking that he be held without bail," the ADA says, unprompted.

I look at him and then at the dock, where the defendants in custody are supposed to stand. There's nobody there. I can't figure out who he is referring to. But I stay quiet. I don't want to look like an idiot.

"Okay," the judge says. "We'll give it a further call so Attorney Nastasia can go down and talk to her client."

Holy shit, I think. *Down is where the lockup is.* My already fast-beating heart pounds in my chest and my palms are sweating. I don't even know where to start. Andrea, the lawyer I'm shadowing, is still nowhere to be found.

"Here's the complaint and police report," a court officer says as he hands me a packet of paperwork. "You can get his record from probation." He points his chin toward the probation desk to my left as he speaks.

"Thank you," I say out loud. And to myself—*thank God.*

With the fourteen-page criminal record of my new client in hand, I sit at one of the back tables to read the police report before going to the lower level to meet with him.

As I walk down the stairs, I practice saying the word "recognizance" in my head, reciting it over and over so I won't screw it up during the hearing.

Marshall is easy to find; he's the only one in lockup.

"Hi. I'm Gail Nastasia. I'm going to be representing you. It's nice to meet you."

"Hi," he says. "Don't worry about trying to get me out of here. I already know that's not happening."

"Probably not since you're already on probation. And the prosecutor asked the judge to hold you without bail."

"And my record ain't pretty. I do crazy shit when I'm using."

If he only knew. "Lots of people do."

"I've cleaned up a few times over the years, but I'm an addict."

I don't tell him I know exactly how he feels, that I'll be celebrating four years clean myself in a few months.

"At least if I'm locked up, I won't have to worry about it for a while."

I can't argue with that.

I head back upstairs to wait for his case to be called.

MY CLIENT SITS quietly in the dock while waiting to hear his name, looking so docile it's hard to believe he's the same guy whose record I'm holding in my lap. Of course, I know how different people can be from what they seem.

When the clerk calls his case, my client struggles to his feet, the leg shackles and handcuffs loosely securing him, and shuffles to the railing. I stand a few feet away, on the other side of the dark wood pony wall that separates us.

The judge turns to the ADA. "Are you asking for bail?"

"Judge, this guy should be held without bail!" he yells, turning to my client. He points toward the dock. "This piece of trash shouldn't be allowed to walk the streets!"

I don't move. I can't move. I'm stunned by his sudden outburst. They didn't teach this in training.

I'm still frozen, wondering whether they're all in on it, playing some kind of practical joke on the new girl, when I hear a ruckus to my left.

"Fuck you, you pussy. I'll kill you!" my client screams back as he tries to climb over the barrier that separates him from the rest of us. My stomach clenches as I take an instinctive step to my right, away from him. He reminds me of the angry, drunken men of my childhood, and I feel like a kid again.

A few seconds later, three court officers are on him, pulling him from the railing and onto the floor. And then he's gone.

"See, judge? He's an animal," the ADA says.

My head snaps in his direction. Although I'm still reeling from the surprise of what's just happened, I can see that this was no joke. He baited my client. The ADA manipulated the situation, knowing full well he'd react the way he did.

I inhale and open my mouth, ready to tell the judge just that, but I don't say anything. I'm new here, and I don't want to get on anybody's bad side. The bigger truth is that I have way more in common with my client than I do with these men. And at the moment, I'm more afraid of them than I am of him.

"Okay, Attorney Nastasia," the judge says. "Mr. Jones is going to be held without bail. Let's pick a thirty-day date for his next appearance."

Now that I have an actual court date in my schedule, I'll have to figure out the procedure for a jail visit.

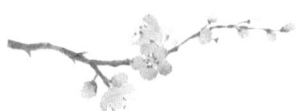

11

HOUSE OF CORRECTION

With the exception of some fresh paint and new waiting room benches, the county jail lobby looks exactly the same as it did fifteen years ago, when I visited my then boyfriend, Jack. But being here in my capacity as an attorney feels completely different than when I used to come as a regular visitor.

From where I'm standing, waiting to go through the metal detector, I can see most of the large, brightly lit room. It's littered with more than a dozen people. There's another smaller room that sits just beyond the conveyor belt. At the moment, it holds a corrections officer who's checking people in. Beside it, there's a small desk and a third CO.

The line shrinks quickly. When it's my turn, I put the plastic bin containing my client file, car keys, pen, and credentials on the belt. This is my second time through—I made the rookie mistake of bringing my purse the first time. I thought they'd have lockers for lawyers, but they don't. I had to leave my valuables in my car like everybody else.

This time, I've done everything right. I have only the necessities. Still, when the machine beeps as I move through the metal detector, my neck tightens, and my breath catches on its way out. I'm not doing anything wrong or carrying any contraband, but my nervous system doesn't seem to know I'm not the young drug-addicted girl I was when I was here last.

I look at the officer, who gestures with his left hand for me to come forward. There's a wand in his right hand.

"Arms out," he says, all business.

I try to lighten the moment with small talk as he waves the wand over my body. "I didn't realize it was visiting hours. I would've waited an hour."

The beeping increases when the wand passes over my waist.

"The schedule is online," he says with disinterest.

"Yeah, thanks. I think it's my belt." I'm starting to sweat, and my heart is beating so fast I feel like it might push right through my chest.

"You're good," he says finally. "Check in over there." He points his chin toward the only desk without plexiglass.

I attempt to steady my breathing as I collect my things and make my way further into the room, following the guy's direction.

"Visitor's slip?" the uniformed man behind the desk says without looking up.

"No, I'm not sure what I'm supposed to do. I'm an attorney."

He lifts his head, his eyes meeting mine, "Oh. You haven't been here before?"

"No," I say without hesitation. "I'm new at this." I smile and hold his gaze despite my urge to turn away. I don't tell him I've been here several times, because then I'll have to tell him why.

"Oh, okay." His smile is a relief. "You don't need to fill out a slip, just put your name in this book and list who you're here to see on one of those sheets," he says, pointing at a pad on the counter. "Then put it in that drawer with your bar card and ID."

Shit, my ID. It suddenly occurs to me that they might figure out who I am. Yes, my last name is Nastasia, but I'm still the same Gail Brenner who's visited here—and many other prisons—all those years ago. My social security number hasn't changed.

I wonder if I look as sketchy as I feel—like I'm an imposter pretending to be somebody important.

"And I'll take your car keys," he says, holding out his hand.

"Thank you," I say in my most grateful, relaxed voice as I hand them over.

I take my time signing the attorney log book and filling out the other sheet. I'm in no rush to hand over my license. What if they look me up and tell me I'm not allowed to come here? If I can't come to the jail, I won't be able to do my job, and I can't change my answer about not having been here before; I've already lied.

When I run out of ways to delay the inevitable, I drop the form, my bar card, and my license into the open drawer and watch as it disappears, the drawer front becoming flush with the wall. For a moment, I just stand there, thinking the drawer might slide back out right away. When it doesn't, I turn to find a place to sit.

Leaning against the wall of windows, I look for an empty spot. The long ten-or-so metal benches are occupied mostly by women and girls and a few children. One of the twenty-ish looking women is holding an infant; she reminds me of myself at that age, waiting to see Jack.

Jack was my whole world back then, when the jail was still shiny and new. He was the man who played peek-a-boo with baby Alita and promised we'd be together forever. I promised to stay by his side as we faced his legal troubles. Catching a case wasn't a big deal, I told him. There wasn't a single person I knew, including me, who hadn't had run-ins with the law.

On my first prison visit to see Jack, I'd stood in a lobby much like this one, terrified they'd discover my prior arrests and turn me away. When the guard handed my ID back that day, I'd nearly collapsed with relief.

But this visit is different. I'm different. Still, the fear feels exactly the same.

Tap tap tap. The sound jars me back into the room. When I turn to its source, I see an officer who's standing behind the glass, pointing to the receiver next to the drawer. I pick it up.

"Have you been here before?"

Shit. He must've found something. I can see him looking at the computer screen. I double down. "No," I say, my throat dry.

"Alright, well, this might take a while."

After replacing the receiver, I walk to the window for a glimpse of the outside. The weather is perfect on this early spring Wednesday; everything brown is beginning to turn green. But I can't see it from here. Most of what is visible from the window is man-made—the parking lot and a building next door. Even from here though, there are signs of what's beyond this place: green grass, trees, and the light blue sky. Freedom. I wonder how these guys handle being locked in a cell when I can't manage less than half an hour in the lobby. Of course, it's not like they have any choice.

I walk back toward the desk where I filled out the paperwork, and then to the window again. And back to the desk. I'm pacing, sweating. I need a moment alone. I look to the door marked with a "W", and as much as I don't want to use the bathroom in this place, it's my only option for privacy.

I'm embraced by quiet when the door to the single-stall bathroom closes behind me. I turn the lock, careful to breathe through my mouth just in case it smells bad. Now that I'm alone, the tension drains from my neck and shoulders like water through a colander. I close my eyes and roll my head all the way around, giving my muscles the stretch they so badly need during this momentary reprieve. I'm not free and clear yet.

Balancing my file on the corner of the sink, I wash my hands and dry them under the low heat of the electric wall unit. The dryer is so slow that even though I'm in no rush to leave my solitude, I reach for the toilet paper instead.

Back in the lobby, I find a seat at the end of a bench closest to the room where my future is currently under review. If I were a praying person, I would probably do that now. I've softened to the idea a little, but I'm far from convinced it would make any difference. Since there's nowhere to look without appearing to be nosey, I open my client's file and begin reading through the police report again, even though I've read it so many times, I could recite it from memory.

At least twenty minutes have passed when the drawer finally slides open.

"You're all set," the guy yells through the space. "Sorry for the wait. Next time, try to come when it's not regular visiting hours."

I smile and swipe the contents from the drawer before he can take them back. "Thank you," I say, clipping the visitor badge to my lapel.

As I move toward the door, muscle memory kicks in—I already know the way. This time though, instead of joining the crowd that will head to plexiglass visits, I go through the door alone and wait in the vestibule. When the second door opens, I move through it as though I've done it a hundred times, my heels clicking against the pavement as I walk past the barbed wire. This time, I open the door on the left where the sign says "Attorney Visits."

At the end of the hall, through another unlocked door, I have my first glimpse of the attorney-visiting area where my client and I will meet in private.

As I wait for Marshall alone in the room that's just big enough for a small table and a few chairs, I remember how just two days ago, he tried to attack the prosecutor. If he has a similar outburst today, I'll be trapped in this compact space with him. Although my insides are shaking, I do my best to hold it together. This is my job.

I stand and extend my hand when he enters. He smiles and shakes my hand. "Thank you for coming," he says, as though I'm his houseguest. He's the same calm man I met in lockup, not the one he became in the courtroom, and the hour-long meeting is a success.

Once I'm back in the comfort of my Jeep, I breathe in deep and smile. I did it. After all that work, I pulled it off. I wish my mother could see me now. She'd be proud. I know exactly what she would say: "I never doubted you for a second."

2007-2008

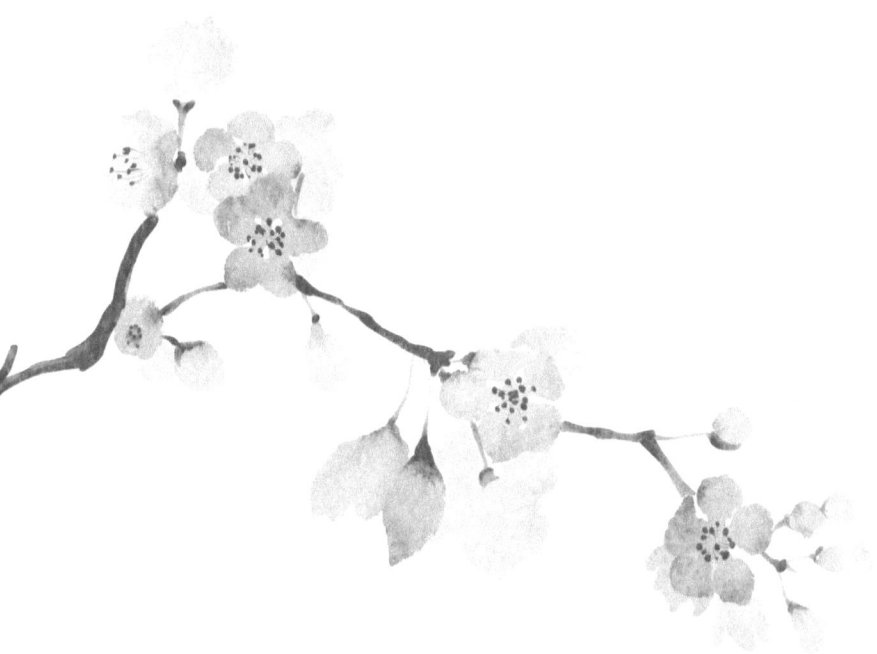

12

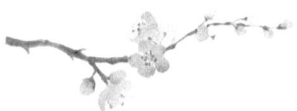

LINEAGE

"Where do you want us?" Pam asks, looking over the cardboard boxes stacked on the dining room table. Of all the wives, Pam is the most outspoken, which makes her most like me. Joann stands beside her, to my right, and Kathy is a few feet away, leaning against the sparkling black granite of the kitchen peninsula. Our husbands are busy moving furniture from the other house.

The women look at me expectantly, waiting for instructions on how to unpack our new house. I look around the room; I have no idea where to start. All these things are new to me—home, supportive friends, normalcy.

"The china cabinet," I say finally, as though I know exactly how to conduct this orchestra of help. I've been secretly waiting to dress this cupboard for months. The idea of filling it gives me hope for my future here. From the very first time I walked through the house alone, I knew it was my chance to give my kids the home I never had.

That day, after unlocking the front door, I stood in the foyer, taking it all in. Then, I gave myself a tour of our new home. The place was a mess. It had been an estate sale, and the owner's brother had lived here alone for several years. According to the owner, his brother was married when he bought the place and had intended it to be his dream home. He added state-of-the-art kitchen appliances and raised the roof to make room for kids that would never come. When his wife left him and the house, the work ended, but he stayed here alone.

After walking through the entire house, downstairs and up, I ended right here in the dining room. I stood in this same spot, looking at the cabinet, its dust-covered glass doors, imagining what it could be. It reminded me of my mother, and how when she was drug-free, bright-eyed, and full of dreams, convinced that she'd beat heroin, she'd lead Chrissy and me through each new apartment, pointing out all the things she loved about the place. In one apartment, I remember her standing in the living room, gazing at what I thought was a dresser.

"Look at these built-ins," she said, her eyes filled with promise. Being in that moment made me feel a sense of stability, rare for our family, as three years was the longest we lived anywhere.

I thought about all my temporary places—the foster homes, shelters, and my apartment rentals. Back when I never knew how long I'd be able to stay in one home or another, I couldn't imagine I'd ever own a home. People like me and my siblings, who grew up in addiction and poverty, didn't have the money or resources it takes to own property.

But now I have my own built-ins. I can create the security my mother couldn't and build the foundation she talked about when I was a teenager; the one she said had to be strong enough to support a family.

That's exactly what I plan to do. And not just for me and my kids, but for Chrissy and Philip too. It'll be good for all of us to have a place to come together as a family. I smile at the thought of it.

I open one of the boxes on the table in front of me, lift out one of the flat, newspaper-wrapped objects, and pull the paper away as though I'm opening a delicate gift. Inside is a plate with gold rimming the edge and flowing across the top in an intricate floral design. It feels light in my hands, smooth except for the embossed pattern. I run my fingers over the large pink rose in the center, surrounded by forest green leaves and blue, yellow, and purple flowers.

"Oh, that's so pretty," Pam says, leaning in for a closer look. Joann and Kathy do the same before they each pull their own piece from the box. They start unwrapping the rest of the pieces, wiping away the dust that has worked its way through the paper's protection over the years. "Where did you get it?"

"Ronnie's mother."

"That was nice," Kathy says. She's right, of course. But the gesture still surprises me. In the seven years since Ronnie and I met, Mary and I have had only a handful of conversations. I'm not even sure she likes me.

The day Mary offered me the set, we'd gone to Ronnie's parents' apartment for more renovation money, cash that Tom called a "loan." Mary stepped out of the room and returned a few minutes later with a small cardboard box. She removed one of its contents and unwrapped a dainty teacup.

"Do you want these?" she asked as she handed it to me. "It's a twelve-piece set."

It was the third time she'd handed me a gift; the first was a five-hundred dollar check at my baby shower for Serena, and the second was a gold pendant of the scales of justice on the day I became a lawyer.

As I cradled the fragile cup, I was struck by the gravity of her offering. While I know little about lineage and pedigree or how the dynamics of a real family work, I fully understood that Mary could have given her collection to her other daughter-in-law, the wife of Ronnie's brother, but she chose me. This was exactly what my new built-in had been waiting for.

"Of course," I managed, my throat tightening at the gesture. Maybe she was coming to see me as part of the family, and this was her way of welcoming me in. I couldn't imagine using such formal dinnerware, but, yes, more than anything, I wanted the set.

I turn to the cabinet behind me, its shelves now clean and bare, ready to welcome these beautiful pieces to their new home. I place the first plate on the second shelf, but something doesn't look right—the design can't be seen from this angle. There has to be a better way. I lean the plate against the back wall, then quickly realize there's nothing to stop it from sliding down. After placing another freshly polished plate at its base for support, it seems stable enough, but the arrangement looks crude and unrefined. I stare at the awkward display, completely at a loss for how to make this work.

"This is not my forte," I say to the women, my tone light as I step aside.

Without missing a beat, the three of them take over. Kathy, who has a way with design, positions herself in front of the cabinet and places each piece meticulously inside, as if following some invisible blueprint. Pam and Joann hand the dishes to her, all of them working seamlessly as a team.

Watching from the sidelines, I feel the familiar weight of being on the outside. Although these women seem to have accepted me into their group, I'm not quite sure I belong. They move with an easy confidence I don't possess, handling things that feel foreign to me as naturally as breathing.

I slip away, into the kitchen where the boxes of regular plates are. I know how to unpack those.

With so many helping hands, the unpacking goes quickly. A few hours after our guests arrived, they say their goodbyes and leave our small family in our new home.

Once Serena and Ronnie are in bed, I embrace my time alone. I go back downstairs, again taking my time as I move through the first floor, noticing even the smallest details. I'm proud of the work I've done here, laying tile and painting walls.

At the back door, I flip on the light and open one of the side panels, letting in the warm August air and the chirping and peeping of wetland creatures. To me, it sounds like music.

I turn off the light and walk back into the dining room, where I pause before the cabinet. It looks stunning, the heirlooms of my husband's family arranged by his friends—our friends. This is my home. It is entirely possible that I fit here with Ronnie, in this house, on this street, and in this world. From where I'm standing, everything looks perfect.

13

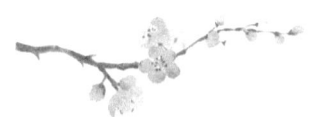

THE ESCAPE ARTIST

Thankfully, Jack is on babysitting duty tonight. It's my women's meeting night, and if there was ever a time when I needed a meeting, it's now. I've been so overwhelmed since the move to the new house, and this is exactly what I need. Although I keep reminding myself I should be grateful, that the days of doing it all on my own are in the past, the pressure is crushing me.

At 6:45, I grab my purse from the kitchen counter and yell goodbye to the kids. The meeting starts at seven. I'm halfway out the door before realizing my travel mug is still on the counter. It's just a few steps away, and since I only meant to grab it and go, I leave the door ajar. That's all it takes. Rocco, our rottweiler bolts through the opening, seizing his chance at freedom.

"Shit," I say under my breath, so Serena won't hear it upstairs. Now I'll have to get him back inside before I leave. Jack can't help; he has to stay with Serena. And Ronnie is already at his meeting, which is probably a good thing. Rocco getting out has been the source of many arguments between us lately.

I put my cup on the counter and walk out onto the front stoop, where I call his name. A few seconds later, he appears in the driveway, panting, his tongue wagging the way his tail would if he had one.

"Come on, Rocco," I say, in the sweetest, most cheerful tone I can muster. He takes a few steps in my direction before breaking right, running in front of the garage doors, and disappearing into the darkness. I can't tell whether he's gone behind the house or through the side yard and into the neighbor's yard. Even if it were daylight, I'd never be able to catch him.

IT'S HARD TO believe this is the same dog who brought us all such joy two Christmases ago when I surprised Ronnie with the puppy. I knew how happy he'd be since he had to put Harley, the dog he had when we met, down a few years before Serena was born.

After opening presents that morning, Alita and Jack met my friend Wendy at the back gate and snuck the pooch into the house. They returned to the living room a few minutes later with a big box.

"This is for you," Alita said.

When the box moved, Ronnie smiled big. As he lifted one of the flaps, Rocco's furry head popped up. Serena laughed and toddled over to get a closer look.

"Oh my God," Ronnie said, his grin so wide his eyes crinkled.

"This is Rocco," I said, having already chosen the name. It was what Ronnie had wanted to call Serena if she'd been a boy.

Ronnie leaned forward, and gripping the puppy under his front legs, lifted him out of the box and held him high above his head to get a good look. "Hey, Rocco," he said, laughing. Then we took pictures of our happy family, one with Ronnie holding Rocco in one arm and Serena in the other. Thinking of it now, I can't even muster a smile.

As much as I want to get in my Jeep and drive away, pretending that I don't know he's out there running around in the dark, I can't bring myself to do it. I text Ronnie, "Rocco's out. You really need to put up that electric fence." I wish I could tell him the truth, that I'm struggling, but I'm not one to show weakness.

My eyes fill with tears for the second time today. The stress of these last few months is too much, but even more than that, I can't figure out why I'm having so much trouble handling it. I was a single parent who managed everything by myself for twelve years before meeting Ronnie. I got the kids to school, made sure they had full bellies and clean clothes, and paid the bills—all while attending college. The only help I had was through welfare and food stamps. Now that I have somebody to share the burden, this should be easy.

"Please," I whisper into the dark. But I know that even if Rocco could hear, he wouldn't listen to me. He doesn't respect me. Never has. I learned that lesson at the old house when he was still a puppy.

That night, over a year ago, I'd let him out to go to the bathroom. It was ten o'clock and pitch black outside. He didn't come when I called him back in, so I went out into the yard. Being as dark as the night, I didn't see Rocco coming until right before he jumped on me, knocking me to the ground. Every time I tried to pull myself to my feet, he'd jump on me again, wrestling me back down. At nearly one hundred pounds, he weighed almost as much as I did, and he was so much stronger than me. As loud as I screamed for Ronnie, who was sound asleep on the other side of the wall, he didn't hear.

A good twenty minutes passed before I was finally able to escape Rocco and get back into the house. Since then, I've had little to say about what he does. And now that he's over two years old, I doubt that will ever change.

I walk to the side yard and then out back. Standing in the grass, I listen for a splash or a bark, but all I hear are the nighttime critters playing their orchestra. Then, with my hands on my hips, I yell his name into the dark wetlands that butt up against our property. On other nights, I've worried about him getting stuck in the muddy water, but tonight I'm too exasperated to care. He isn't back here.

After a few minutes of calling into the void, I go back inside for my purse and try the driving-around approach instead. For the next ten minutes, I drive in circles, hoping to catch sight of him, but at this point, I'm not even sure I want to find him.

Finally, I give up and drive to Kate's house where the meeting has already started. Although I've managed to steady my breathing, I'm still on edge as I drag a chair from the kitchen into the living room to join the other six ladies.

"You're late," Kathy says.

I know she's joking, but I'm in no mood to play along. "I know. Rocco got out again. I drove around the neighborhood looking for him for half an hour, but he was nowhere to be found. He'll come home when he wants."

"You just left him outside?" Pam asks with wide eyes.

I don't even try to stop the tears. Her confirmation of my inadequacy is more than I can bear. My hands move to cover my face instinctively; I've always hated the ugly way I look when I cry. And the women, all of them seated around the room, are watching me.

"Oh no, I'm sorry. Don't cry," Pam says.

Now that she feels bad, I feel even more guilty for causing a scene, which makes me cry even more.

"I don't know what to do," I say between short breaths. "I feel trapped. I keep telling Ronnie that he has to do something—at least walk the dog. Maybe if he got some exercise, he wouldn't run for the door whenever it's opened. And I can't walk him. He's so strong that he ends up walking me. I've even threatened to find Rocco a new home if Ronnie won't take care of him. He just says he will. But he still hasn't put up the electric fence Bert gave us. It's sitting in a dining room drawer waiting to be installed." I'm rambling.

"Maybe Bert can come over and help put it in," Kathy says. She and her husband are always willing to help us out.

"It'll get better," Pam says. "He's still a puppy."

They're just trying to help, but nothing they say is making me feel any better. What I won't tell them, or anybody for that matter, is that I wish I'd never gotten Rocco to begin with. Having a dog is so much work. I have a hard enough time taking care of humans.

I take a deep breath and wipe my eyes. "Day at a time," I say, attempting a smile. They must recognize my desire to move on, because that's what we do. Despite there being no resolution, for the moment at least, I'm not in the middle of the mess.

ROCCO IS INSIDE when I get home. I pat his head when he runs to the door; I'm trying not to be resentful toward him. I know it's not his fault.

I find Ronnie upstairs, lying in bed watching television. "Hey," he says, as though the day has been business as usual.

"Hey," I say before going into the bathroom and shutting the door behind me.

As I wash my face and brush my teeth, I'm trying to figure out how to approach Ronnie with what I'm feeling in a way that won't cause a fight. I get why he thinks the way he does—in his mind, his parents had it figured out. His mother took care of the house and kids while his father paid the bills. Clean division of labor. But we're not his parents. His mother didn't split her time between taking care of the house, kids, and clients who depended on her. And unlike Ronnie's mother, I bring home a paycheck, which means if we're sharing the bills equally, the household responsibilities should be divided the same way.

I dry my hands, open the door, and start talking as I walk toward him.

"I'm really overwhelmed. It's hard to keep up with everything." I sit on my side of the bed.

"Do we really have to have this conversation right now?"

"Yeah. We hardly see each other during the week."

"It's almost ten," he says. "I have to get up at five-thirty."

"I know, but something has to change. I was in tears trying to get Rocco back in the house earlier. You have to help more. I can't do everything." I take a deep breath, and wait for a new threat of tears to pass.

"Yeah, well I have my job."

"I know, Ronnie. I have a job too."

"No kidding. But you work for yourself, and I don't."

We've been having the same argument for over a month. No matter what I say, it always ends up in the same place. "Kathy said she'd ask Bert to help install the electric fence."

"Fine. I'll do it this weekend."

The way he says it, like he's doing me a favor, makes me want to scream— *Rocco is your dog, and Serena is also your daughter!* But I don't. That'll only keep the fight going. Instead, I get under the covers, switch off my side-table lamp, and wait for the sweet relief of sleep.

14

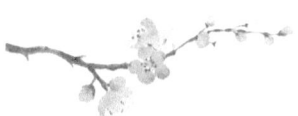

NURTURER

Serena didn't wake up on her own this morning like she usually does. I found her in bed with a runny nose and bright pink cheeks.

"Aw, sweetie. You stay here. I'll get you a drink and a cool facecloth for your head."

Downstairs in the kitchen, I dialed Ronnie, who had already gone to work.

"Serena's sick. She feels hot too. I'm pretty sure she's got a fever, although I haven't checked yet."

"Are you bringing her to Vilma's?"

"I can't bring her there if she's sick. Vilma's got five other kids she has to keep healthy." But he knows that already. "You're going to have to come home and stay with her while I go to court."

"What are you talking about? I can't just take off work."

"I'll be as quick as I can, probably an hour or two."

"I have shit to do. You'll have to call out," he said matter-of-factly.

"Ronnie, I can't call out. My client is in jail, and if I don't show up, he'll have to stay there even longer." Wilson is an addict like me, who's only stuck behind bars because he can't make the two-hundred-dollar cash bail.

"I don't know what to tell you," he said. "Check her temperature. Maybe she doesn't have a fever, and you can bring her to Vilma's."

There was no point in arguing with him. He's stubborn, especially when it comes to his routine. He's always been that way.

But despite his unwillingness to change, everything else has. We have so many more responsibilities than we did six years ago, when Alita, Jack, and I first moved into Ronnie's house. Back then, the four of us quickly eased into a groove. Ronnie managed his asbestos removal crew, while I handled the bulk of my old friend Peter's bankruptcy practice at home. Alita and Jack, although still young at ten and thirteen, were self-sufficient in many ways. They could get themselves ready for school and find snacks on their own when they got home. We'd order out for dinner most nights, since neither Ronnie nor I like to cook, and share in the clean-up.

Now, though Alita is living with her father, Jack is still with us and in high school, and we have Serena. And as much as I love being in our new house, my forever home, it's a lot. I'm afraid that if Ronnie won't bend, I'll break.

"Thanks for your help," I said calmly, despite the lump in my throat and heat in my face. I hoped he'd hear the frustration in my voice that lay beneath the sarcasm, and tell me he was on his way home, but there was only silence. I closed my eyes and bit the inside of my cheek. If I had time to waste, I would've sat down on one of the high stools tucked against the counter and cried.

I put the phone down, filled a cup with water for Serena, and looked toward the screen again. As hard as I wished he'd call back, my phone stayed dark. *It isn't fair*, I told myself on the way back up the stairs carrying supplies. But as my mother used to say, "Life isn't fair." Nobody was coming to help.

AS IT TURNED out, Serena didn't have a fever. I was able to drop her off at daycare and get to court just a few minutes late. She felt better when I picked her up.

Now, she's playing in her room, and I'm sitting at my desk on the second floor foyer marking off each bill I've paid so far this month. I recently inherited this new bill-paying responsibility. I didn't want the job, but Ronnie wasn't doing it right.

The task shift happened last month after I opened the Home Depot bill marked "Past due." That one was supposed to be his responsibility. When I confronted him about it, he said he'd only paid what he could afford, not the full minimum payment. I tried to explain that partial payments still count as late and hurt our credit, but that didn't change his mind. Instead, he said, "Fine. If you think you can do a better job, you pay the bills."

So, I took it over. I created an Excel spreadsheet for our twenty-seven monthly expenses. Each week, Ronnie deposits a set amount into our joint "house" account, and I make sure the bills are paid in full and on time. If I need to pay more than my share, that's what I do.

Looking at the spreadsheet makes my heart beat fast and my breathing shallow. An unavoidable stress-response, I suppose. It's also the end of the month, which means a whole new set of bills will come due soon, making my anxiety even worse. This is not how I pictured my life.

Lately, Ronnie's only been adding to my stress. I'm glad he's already gone to his meeting. I've been feeling angrier by the day, and those are the kind of feelings that make me wish for relief.

I sit back in my chair and suck in enough air to fill my lungs. I hold it for as long as I can, while reminding myself of the saying, "A grateful heart will never drink," or in my case, get high. That certainly wouldn't help the situation.

As I exhale, I hear Ronnie's voice cut through the quiet. "You killed him! You killed my fucking dog!" It's coming from outside.

I jump up, and as I start down the stairs, the door swings open.

Ronnie rushes inside. "Rocco's dead! He killed him!" He's still standing in the doorway, his eyes wild, as he points outside. When I reach him, I can see a small white car that's idling in the street in front of our house.

"What do you mean? What's happening?" I keep my voice low, hoping Serena, who is still upstairs in her room, is too occupied to hear the commotion.

A second later, Serena appears on the stairs. She stands motionless, waiting for him to say more. I'm sure she's as surprised as I am. Neither of us has ever heard her father sound this way.

Ronnie doesn't acknowledge Serena as he walks into the kitchen, where he stands for a moment, then paces back toward the foyer.

"What happened?" I ask again. Rocco can't be dead. He left the house less than twenty minutes ago, and Ronnie has a tendency to exaggerate.

"That asshole hit him!" he yells. His voice cracks. "He came speeding around the fucking corner!"

"Who?" I ask, but he's already walking toward the door. "I'll be right back, sweetie," I say as I follow him out, carefully closing the door behind me so Serena won't join us.

I stay close behind Ronnie as he walks in the direction of his truck, which is haphazardly parked alongside the stone wall that marks our property line. I'm fast on his heels, my bare feet slapping against the asphalt. The white car is still pulled to the side of the road like it's waiting for somebody to come out, but it's facing the wrong direction. The headlights are on, and although they cut through the darkness, I can't see Rocco or any evidence that he's been hit.

"You killed my dog! I can't fucking believe you did this!" Ronnie yells again at a young kid standing next to the car's rear bumper. He looks like a high-schooler.

"It's not my fault. He came running out into the street. I didn't have time to stop."

I hear the front door open and turn to see Serena's silhouette in the sliver of light from the doorway. Worried she'll come outside, I run back to the house.

When I close the door, she looks up at me, her eyes filled with worry. "Why's Daddy yelling?" She waits for an answer.

"Something happened."

"Is Rocco dead?" It seems unnatural to hear the harsh, blunt sound of the word come from her lips. At four, I know she's only parroting her father, that she doesn't know what it means to be dead, but her curiosity requires me to say something.

"I don't know. I'm still trying to figure out what's going on. Why don't you go upstairs and play, and I'll be up soon." She does as I say, but I can see that she's confused. I'll need to tell her something soon.

I'm in the dining room when Ronnie opens the door a few minutes later.

"I have to go bring him to the vet's," he says as he charges into the room.

"Oh. Okay. Do you think he's going to be all right?" I ask, pulling out a dining room chair.

"No. He's not going to be all right. He's dead. I put him in the back of my truck," he says, sounding angry. If I didn't know him so well, I'd think he was being sarcastic.

Words escape me. I'm terrible at expressing sympathy. All I can think to do is to offer Ronnie a hug, but since he's not ready to be consoled, the embrace is quick and awkward.

When he leaves, the house is quiet again.

I sit at the table and wonder what to do next. Rocco is gone. Of course, it was only a matter of time since there was no barrier to keep him out of the street. Part of me feels relieved that I won't have to worry about him anymore, and that makes me feel even worse. I want to cry, but I hear Serena on the stairs.

A moment later, she's standing in front of me, our eyes at the same level. "Where's Rocco?" she asks.

"Daddy is bringing him to the doctor."

"Why?"

"He ran into the street and was hit by a car."

"Will the doctor make him better?"

"I don't think so, honey. We probably won't be able to see him again." I'm not sure how much of what's happening she can understand, although she's always seemed wise beyond her years.

She looks at me intently, her blue-green eyes big and searching. "Why can't I see him?" She can't remember a time when he didn't live with us.

"I think he's going to heaven."

She looks away, the tip of her pinky touching her top lip like Dr. Evil in *Austin Powers*, a self-soothing habit she's had her whole life.

"I'm hungry," she says. I'm glad she doesn't ask me anything else. Although I've been dealing with loss and death my whole life, nobody ever explained it to me. I have no idea how to explain it to her. I guess that means I'm about as good at nurturing as I am at sympathy, but I can only do my best.

I reach for her, and she wraps her arms around my neck.

"I'll make you some pizza rolls."

15

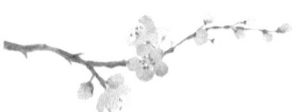

BALL DROP

So far, this has been the best Christmas ever. Lying here with a full belly, listening to the sounds of my family, I can't think of anything better.

It's moments like these that make it easy to be grateful. This year has been such a crazy ride. Rocco's death was hard, and it's taken several months to adjust to being here without him, but we're healing. And despite the problems between Ronnie and me, we're still doing this life thing together.

Things are so good, it's almost as if those early years, when I was a homeless teen with nowhere to go, never happened at all. Back then, while people were spending time with their families, it had been my loneliest time of the year. Those days are behind me.

Today has been perfect, right from the start. Even though I was up late wrapping presents—I've never been one to plan well enough ahead to get it all done before Christmas Eve—I felt well rested and ready for the day.

Ronnie was in the bathroom when I went downstairs to stuff the turkey and put it in the oven. I made my tea, and sat next to the pellet stove to sip it, feeling warm and happy. I knew Serena would be up early. She stayed up late too, waiting for Santa to arrive. Being four now, she knows exactly what Christmas is all about.

Alita arrived by eight-thirty for gift-opening. When she moved in with her father, I worried we wouldn't spend much time together, but she's been here for both Christmases in this house. Having all my kids in the same place is the best part of the day.

We sat around the tree: me on the recliner, Ronnie on the couch, and the kids on the floor. Except for Alita, we all wore pajamas, our hair messy from sleep.

As Alita and Jack handed out gifts, I remembered what Christmas was like for me as a kid. We rarely had a tree, and our presents were donations given by Globe Santa or some other non-profit organization. What I want most is to give my kids a better experience than I had. As I looked around the room at their smiling faces, I was sure I'd done just that.

Serena giggled as she opened each new toy. Jack tore the paper from his yearly updated Guinness Book of World Records. Alita smiled as she ran her hand over a new leather-covered journal for her collection.

Soon we each had a stack of gifts: sneakers, clothes, video games, books, and for Serena, the Easy-Bake oven I'd wished for as a kid. Next came the stockings. That's where I'd put Ronnie's big gift—a flight to New York City and a two-night stay in Times Square for the New Year's Eve Ball Drop. I'd been so excited for him to open it, and his reaction didn't disappoint. His grateful expression reminded me of when he'd seen the box containing Rocco three years before.

After opening presents, Ronnie went to get the leaf for the dining room table, the kids sorted and played with their bounty, and I went to the kitchen to baste the turkey and peel carrots. It's one of the only times of the year that I enjoy cooking.

Late morning, Chrissy and her husband Mike arrived with their kids, Geoffrey and Brady, and Philip, who they picked up on the way. We greeted each other with hugs, like normal families do. Because that's what we've become.

Along with the spinach dip, mashed potatoes, and squash, they brought presents from Aunt Sherry. Aunt Sherry couldn't come this year because she was hosting her own family gathering, picking up Uncle Bobby from the state hospital, and Aunt Julie from her residential home for Christmas dinner. Like me, she wanted to spend the day with her sister and brother.

Chrissy and I opened our identical ugly Christmas sweatshirts from Aunt Sherry, and then went to work in the kitchen sauteing, boiling, and baking. The kids played upstairs while the guys watched television in the next room. It felt like everybody was exactly where they were supposed to be.

An hour later, we all sat down to eat.

Even with the leaf, the table wasn't big enough for all of us. Alita and Brady sat at the peninsula.

Mike carved the turkey as we passed around bowls of stuffing, mashed potatoes, and Chrissy's squash.

"Mom, can I have some more cranberry sauce?" Geoffrey asked.

"I want some too," Serena said. Then, "Why does it have lines in it?" she asked.

"Fresh from the can," I said. "That's how we do it in our family." Chrissy, Philip, and I laughed the loudest. It was true enough. Our childhood meals were limited to what was cheap, quick, and easy. I looked at my siblings—little Chrissy with her light brown hair, Philip tall and freckled, and me with my dark hair and eyes—and thought about how remarkable it was that we'd stayed together. Three kids with different fathers, our mother gone before any of us turned thirty, and somehow we'd created a cohesive family unit. Yet another thing to be grateful for.

We knew dinner was over when everybody pushed their plates away and leaned back in their chairs.

The kids went back to playing with their toys, and the adults went to the living room. I joined them on the sectional, but as hard as I tried, I couldn't keep my eyes open. It had to be the tryptophan, I said, before making my way upstairs.

Now, as I lie here, I'm excited for what's coming in the year ahead: Ronnie and I starting off our new year in Manhattan, watching the ball drop, Alita's move to college, and Jack's high school graduation. Serena will start preschool soon, too. There's nothing wrong that I can name. Not one single thing.

Dare I say, I'm happy.

2009

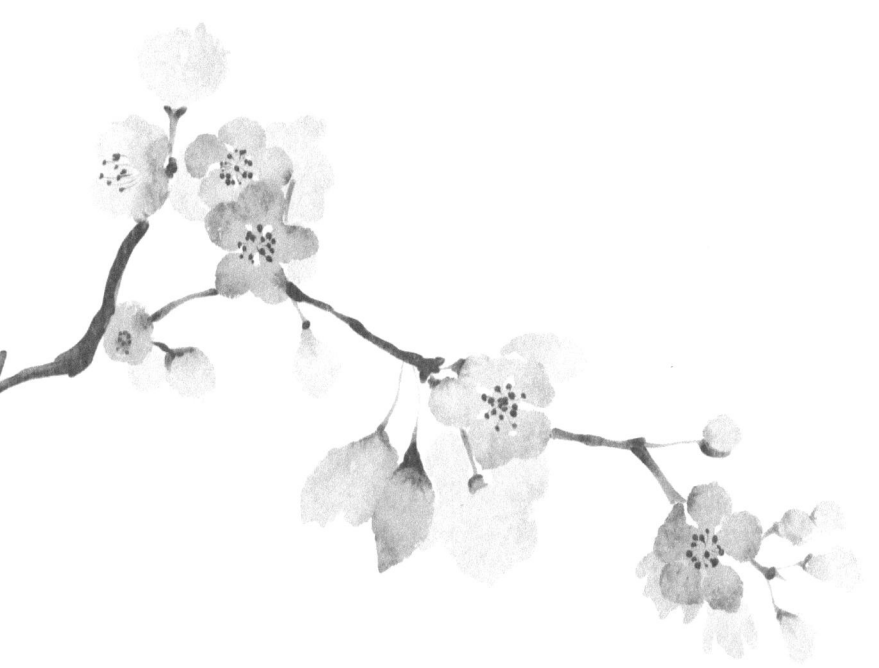

16

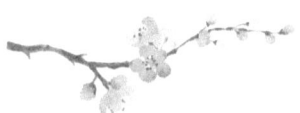

THE MORE THINGS CHANGE...

The new year started off on such a high after the best Christmas of my life. I can't explain what's happened since then. Just a few months into 2009, I'm back to feeling unhappy. What's wrong with me? There's still a ton of outside pressure, but maybe it's true that I just don't know how to be happy.

My default has been to pull away from Ronnie, and look forward to my time alone. Evenings like this have become my refuge.

Tonight, I'm on the living room couch with my laptop. I've just finished writing in my journal, a positive way to deal with my emotions, which I'm trying to make a habit. This week's recording of *American Idol* is playing on the TV as I open Facebook. I'm new to social media, having missed the whole MySpace thing, but I understand immediately that the number hovering over the chat button means I have a message. When I click on it, another window opens.

> *Hey. I ran into a friend of yours and I need to talk to you. I can't explain right now, but you'll understand more when we speak, Chris.*

The words bring with them a rush of heat to my face as I'm immediately transported to 1982, the year I lost my virginity.

Chris.

I've thought about him so many times over the years. Although he didn't turn out to be my first love, or even my boyfriend after we were together that one time, we became friends and hung out on occasion.

The last time I saw Chris was twenty-one years ago. I was seventeen and pregnant with Alita, living on Gloucester's Alper Road, in my very first apartment. Then we lost touch.

I reread the message as I fumble for the remote beside me on the couch. I feel around for the pause button so I don't have to look away from the screen. I listen for the sound of footsteps just in case Ronnie isn't asleep like I thought. Even though I'm not doing anything wrong, I feel like this should be kept secret. The house is quiet.

What could Chris possibly need from me? After all these years? I've heard some things about him, that he'd gotten married and was living on the west coast making lots of money. I wasn't surprised. From what I could remember, Chris was the kind of kid people liked. It didn't hurt that he was good-looking with his dirty-blond mullet, hazel eyes and muscles. But what drew me to him was that he'd been an army brat who, by the time he moved to Gloucester shortly before we met, had already traveled around the world. I loved the idea of going far away.

But none of that was why he was my first. That happened because he was kind to me in a way other boys weren't. He seemed to really like me.

My fingers dance across the keys in response.

Chris?? You sure have surprised the hell out of me. Long time no see. What's going on? How are you? Last I heard, you were living in California.

I look over my shoulder before hitting send.

MY FIRST THOUGHT this morning, as I rubbed sleep from my eyes, was whether Chris had seen my response and if there would be a message waiting for me. I didn't give in to temptation and look right away. I promised myself I'd wait until I was done with court to open the app, but now that I'm here with nothing to do but wait, I can't hold out any longer. I open my laptop on one of the attorney's tables and log in. Nothing.

I feel the immediate embarrassment of rejection. While I keep my eyes trained on the laptop, my focus is on those I can see in my peripheral vision.

I'm wondering whether they noticed the sudden shift in me, how I went from appearing self-assured to full of doubt in a matter of minutes.

Why do I do this to myself? Just when I think I've made progress and I'm not the needy girl I used to be, I'm reminded she's still very much inside of me. I should've ignored the message. I'm married, after all, and according to his Facebook profile, so is Chris. To top it off, I shouldn't be the one who feels rejected—he reached out to me. But of course, I do.

I close my laptop and shove it into my bag. *Screw him.*

THREE DAYS AND still no word from Chris. I haven't stopped thinking about him. That's why I came to my office after court. I want to be alone when I log in to Facebook. Just in case.

I power on my computer before taking my jacket off and hanging it on the back of my chair. As I impatiently wait for the machine to come to life, I run my hand across the smooth leather of my desk pad, a gift from Ronnie. He gave it to me for Christmas along with the Ethan Allen desk it's protecting. He really is a good guy, just not the best partner. Or maybe I'm not the best partner. What do I know?

The computer beeps, and the cursor flashes ready. As per my ritual, I tell myself there won't be a message as a guard against disappointment. It's silly, I know, this attempt to trick myself out of getting my hopes up when there's still no response. But it's what I do.

"Here goes nothing." I slide the mouse, click, and there it is—a message. I hold my breath and click again. It's short:

Can we talk in person? It's private and I could really use your help.

I smile. He hasn't changed his mind. He still needs me. *Of course*, I reply and type my cell phone number.

My phone rings right away. It's an unknown number, and although he didn't say he'd call now, I know it's him. I let it ring twice before answering so I don't appear too eager.

"Law office," I say, my heart pounding.

"Gail?"

"Hey stranger," I say, turning in my office chair, keeping my voice steady.

"It's really you," he says. "I've thought about you so much over the years."

I'm speechless. Of all his possible opening lines, this wasn't one I've considered.

I stand and walk to the window; the nervous energy pulsing through my body needs somewhere to go. "I've thought about you too. How are you?"

"I'll tell you all about it, but first, you're a fucking lawyer!" He sounds impressed not shocked.

"I am," I say, my smile growing wider.

"I'm not at all surprised," he says.

I feel myself stand straighter. I've done such a good job keeping my past out of my present, I didn't know how good it would feel to join the two. Hearing the pride in Chris's voice makes me think maybe there's nothing wrong with me at all. "You must be a little surprised," I say, pushing my hair behind my ear.

"Not a bit," he says. "I always knew you were an extraordinary human." I bite my lip to keep from smiling as I move back toward my desk. Nobody has ever said anything like that to me before. As much as I know Ronnie loves me, he's not big on flattery, and other guys have said I'm pretty and smart. But extraordinary? No. I'm glad he can't see me; I'm sure my cheeks are bright pink.

"Why, thank you," I say, hearing my mother, who would use the same phrase whenever receiving a compliment.

"So, the reason I reached out, is I'm having a problem with pills. I heard you've had some trouble with them yourself, and that you're clean." His admission makes my stomach drop. It's the last thing I expected, and now I feel ridiculous for misreading the situation. I also feel guilty.

"Yeah, I've had my fair share of addiction issues. To say the least," I say, followed by a short, dry chuckle.

"I was hoping you could help me."

"Absolutely," I say. "I'll do whatever I can."

17

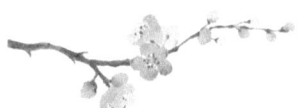

IN MY LIFE

Today's the day. After Chris canceled our first meeting by text, and then canceled again a few days later, I took matters into my own hands. I offered to drive to Gloucester myself. He needed my help, and there was no way I'd bail on him. I'm looking forward to seeing him and, of course, to him seeing me. Especially now that I've finally lost the weight I gained after I quit smoking and then during the pregnancy. I'm almost back down to my twenty-five-year-old size.

Since I'm heading over there right after court, I brought a change of clothes. I want him to see me in my pinstripe suit first, professional and put-together, a far cry from the girl he used to know. Then, I'll change into a fitted blue shirt and jeans so he can really see how good I look.

It's hard to believe it's only been a week since he sent that first message in late March; it feels like it's been a month. Between court, Serena's dance class, and the hundred little things in between, I haven't been able to stop thinking about our upcoming meeting. In my limited spare time, I've been scouring his Facebook page, trying to find out how much he's changed, but his profile picture shows only the mysterious bearded profile of a man wearing a black hat. He was so cute back in our teenage days—all the girls gushed over his long eighties rock star hair and tight jeans. It didn't hurt that he played bass. None of it mattered much to me then. I never saw myself as one of those kinds of girls, and even if I did, Chris didn't see me. Not really. Not in that way.

I keep checking my makeup in the rearview mirror as though something might have changed in the five minutes since I last looked. Damn, I'm nervous.

If I were still a fingernail biter, I'm sure they'd be bleeding by now. And if I were still a smoker, I'd be lighting one off another. As curious and excited as I am, I have no idea what I'm getting myself into. It's been over twenty years since the last time we saw each other, and all I really know is he's got a drug problem.

And on top of the stress of seeing Chris, merely visiting Gloucester is enough to give me heartburn. In the thirteen years since I moved, I do my best to avoid the place. Whenever I do make the forty-five minute drive from home, I start taking deep, calming breaths as soon as the A. Piatt Andrew Bridge is in my sight to keep me from having a panic attack. I try to focus on the beauty of the ocean, which I love, and not the fear. I've been trying to get over it for years, but Gloucester represents a past that I can neither accept nor change. The good news today is that I'm getting off the highway one exit before the bridge. I won't even have to see it.

I PULL ALONGSIDE the curb in front of Chris's business and idle for a few minutes before cutting the engine. I turn the mirror to give myself one last look. This time, I notice the stark contrast between my dark eyebrows and blonde hair. I've been dying my hair this color for over ten years—since before Ronnie and I met—in an effort to reinvent myself. I didn't realize how silly it looked until this very moment. Has it always been this extreme? I suddenly feel like a kid playing dress-up, and I wonder if Chris will think I'm as ridiculous as I feel right now. It doesn't matter; this isn't about me.

Putting the mirror back in place, I take a deep breath and open the door.

Following Chris's directions, I find the second door from the end of the long building and make my way inside. It smells of cigarette smoke and chemicals. I'm facing a hallway and a set of stairs that go down. There are two offices to my left, both of which have open doors. In the office at the front of the building, there's a man sitting behind a very large monitor; all I can see is his tattooed right arm, a lit cigarette in his hand, and the light brown hair on the top of his head. It has to be him.

"Hello?" I say, standing in the doorway just in case I'm wrong and a stranger is sitting behind the desk.

Chris's face appears above the monitor as he stands just tall enough to look over it. There's a telephone wedged between his ear and shoulder. He smiles, holds a finger for me to wait, points to the chair in front of his desk and sits back down. I feel a twinge in my stomach—the gratifying flutter of recognition for the boy I used to know.

I walk to the chair, hook the strap of my pocketbook on its back, and perch on the edge of the seat, shoulders erect, with my bag of clothes in my lap. If anybody were to walk in, they might think I'm here for a job interview.

I'm trying not to eavesdrop as I wait, but I can't help overhearing his conversation about some design project. Although I'm not sure exactly what he does, he sounds experienced and professional. I guess he'd have to be to run his own business. I'm impressed.

I'm also grateful for this chance to ease into the visit and check out the place. Although it could benefit from a deep cleaning, the room is a good size. Even with the desk, chairs, and a filing cabinet on the wall next to where he is sitting, there's still enough space to move around easily. The desk is crowded with empty Dunkin Donut cups and an overflowing ashtray. Behind him, there's a yellow basketball jersey hanging on the wall and a poster of the American Flag with company logos where the stars should be. Photos and what look like kids' drawings are tacked to the wall beside him.

Sitting here, all I can think about is the musty Top of the Harbor basement apartment where Chris and I first met. Gloria's place had been my salvation the summer I turned twelve. It's where I went whenever I needed a respite from the ceaseless fighting between my heroin-addicted mother and her drunken boyfriend. Since Gloria wasn't great at housekeeping, I'd do the dishes just to have somewhere else to be. Quid pro quo.

Besides, her apartment wasn't all that different from the places I'd grown up in. Our apartment at the time, while clean, was overrun with cockroaches and black mold.

Most days, Gloria's living room was filled with us teenagers, guzzling beer or passing a joint around. And when we didn't have something to give us a buzz, we'd play the choking game. One of us would bend over, pant until becoming lightheaded, and then stand up quickly, so another teen could apply pressure to the neck, causing an instant blackout. For me, a few seconds of complete blackness was worth the screaming headache that followed.

Five minutes have passed by the time Chris rolls his chair to his right, away from the monitor's shield, showing me his whole face for the first time in well over a decade. When our eyes meet, a rush of energy flows through my body.

My first thought is that he's even better looking than I remember. His hair is cut above the ears, longer on top instead of the back, unlike the mullet of his past, and he's shaved clean except for a neatly trimmed goatee. His right arm is covered in tattoos, and there are a couple on his left. While I've never thought much about it, the ink looks kind of sexy.

My second thought is that I shouldn't be here.

He rolls back behind the desk.

I feel a sudden urge to move. Where's the bathroom?" I whisper as I stand. "I have to change."

Chris puts his hand over the mouthpiece and lifts his head enough for his eyes to meet mine. "Ask Jess," he says, nodding toward the office next door.

I find his assistant sitting behind her desk. She's pretty, younger than Chris and me, mid-twenties, I guess, and based on the neat stacks of paperwork in front of her, I'm sure she's really the one running things. Still, she doesn't complain about my interruption; she simply stops what she's doing and guides me to the bathroom downstairs.

When I return to Chris's office, he's off the phone. He stands and approaches me with a smile, his arms wide.

"You're here," he says, staring at me as though in disbelief. "It's great to see you." His embrace feels soft and safe, as my cheek presses into his chest.

"It's nice to see you too. It's been a long time."

He takes a step back. "You look fantastic," he says, looking at me as though he's an explorer and I'm uncharted territory. I've never felt so seen.

"Thank you," I manage to say, feeling warmth spread to my face.

"I can't believe you're really here."

"Well, you didn't give me much of a choice. One of us had to do it." We laugh.

"I know. I'm sorry for canceling. Let's get out of here," he says, pocketing the pack of Parliaments that was on his desk.

"Okay, I'll drive," I say, feeling it might be the only thing over which I have any control at the moment. When he scrunches his nose, his eyebrows come together, it's clear he'd rather be the one behind the wheel. But I'm not ready to be his passenger just yet.

"Stage Fort?" I ask, glancing back at him as we move toward the door. "Perfect."

STAGE FORT PARK is mostly empty since it's April, far from high season. In a month from now, when the trees are fully in bloom and the ocean air is warmer, there won't be anywhere to park. But today, I slide right into a space at the beginning of the path to the cannons. That's where we're heading.

Chris and I walk side by side along the shade-covered path; the leaves are nearly in full bloom. The park is quiet, aside from the crunch of gravel under our footsteps. There are a few children playing on the playground to our left, but they too seem subdued, as though respecting this peaceful area.

Despite the path being wide enough for a compact car, we're walking so close our arms touch periodically. I feel a spark of awareness whenever it happens, yet at the same time, I feel more at ease than I have in months.

"This is my favorite place," I say. "Well, so far anyway. It's not like I'm a world traveler. Not yet."

"It's pretty great," Chris says.

"My stepsister Debbie used to bring me here when I was a little kid. She was the only adult who got me away from the insanity at home."

"Yeah, I knew things were fucked up for you."

"I know you know," I say. "Remember that time I came to your house high on Valium, devastated because my boyfriend had been cheating on me? It's hazy, but I recall you guiding me to the brown leather couch where I cried like a baby."

"My parents still have that couch," he says. Again, we laugh.

"And you just listened to me blabber on. Your mother kept poking her head in. I'm sure she was wondering what the hell was going on and hoping you wouldn't leave with me."

"Not at all. She felt bad for you, just like I did. And I wanted to beat the shit out of Jimmy even though I wouldn't have known him if I tripped over him. The thought of it still makes me sick." Of course he doesn't know the half of it. He has no idea what I did for money back then, and I don't plan on telling him.

"But holy shit, look at you now," he steps away as he says it as if to get a better look. And the way his eyes drink me in sends a jolt of heat through my body; like a spark that's ready to burst into flames. This moment makes the trek down my sordid memory lane worth it. "You really are a sight for sore eyes," he says. We're both silent for a moment.

"And you stole my virginity," he smiles.

"You stole mine too," I say, bumping against him.

"Holy shit, remember Gloria's apartment?"

"How could I forget?" Of course I remember the day he showed up—the new kid in town. A week later, we ended up in Gloria's bed. We kissed, took off our pants, and touched each other in private places. I felt lucky that he'd chosen me. But we were over as soon as we left the bedroom. He didn't ask about the next time we'd see each other or if I'd be his girlfriend.

Even after all these years, I can't tell Chris the truth of how I felt back then, or that it still hurts that he didn't want me for more than a few minutes one weekend afternoon. Being honest about the way I feel, no matter how long ago it happened, is damn-near impossible. Instead, I change the subject.

"Gloria's apartment is vivid in my mind, but where she's concerned I draw a complete blank," I say. "Was she ever there?"

"I don't think so. All I know is that being with you that day was one of the best days of my life."

I smile, but don't respond. We shouldn't be having such an intimate conversation.

A few minutes later, he breaks the silence. "So, like I told you on the phone, I'm having some trouble with pills. I started taking them here and there, but now it's out of control. And I really want to stop. I have to stop."

"I know what that's like. I tried for years and failed so many times, I thought I'd never be able to put them down for good."

"You'll help me?"

"Of course."

We walk in comfortable silence, both lost in our own thoughts. The weight of what we've shared hangs between us, but it doesn't feel heavy. To me, it feels like relief. By the time we reach the end of the path where the old cannons point toward the harbor, we're both shivering from the cool ocean air.

"We should head back," he says. "I have a lot to get done, and I've been gone too long already."

"Yeah, I need to get home," I say, although I'd like nothing more than to stay in his company. "Let me know when you want to go to a meeting. I know how hard it is to walk into a room full of strangers. I'll go with you if you want."

"That would be fantastic, Gail. You have no idea how relieved I feel knowing you're in my corner."

We make plans to meet at a Friday night meeting in Gloucester in a few days.

I BLAST THE heat and put the window down as I drive south along Route 128. The spring air is refreshing, and I feel at peace. After all these years, Chris is back in my life.

Just a few minutes into the drive, I hear the familiar opening notes of my favorite Beatles song on the radio, "In My Life." I turn up the volume and sing in harmony with John Lennon. The timing can't be a coincidence, can it? I was just at Stage Fort Park, which reminded me of Debbie, who first introduced me to the Beatles. And I was there with Chris, my first. It all has to mean something.

LATER THAT NIGHT, after everybody is in bed, I log into Facebook. There's a message waiting. My heart races as I click to open it.

> It was so good to see you today. Being with you felt like slipping into my favorite pair of jeans.

His words trigger something deep inside me; an awakening. Reading the message a second time, I feel the same rush of excitement. *Stop it.* It's not right that I feel this way. I close my laptop and put it on the hassock in front of me as though it is the problem. Turning on the television, I try to put Chris and his message out of my mind. But I can't stop thinking about him.

"What's the harm in looking?" I whisper before picking up the offending computer. I read it again before typing:

> It was great to see you too. I'm looking forward to meeting up.

The moment I press send I recognize the feeling I'm having. It's the same rush I'd get when a doctor handed me a prescription for Percocet or when Teddy would call with a fresh batch of Fentanyl patches. But this feels even better than getting high.

18

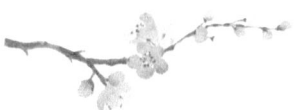

THE KISS

It's Tuesday night, and I haven't seen Chris since Friday afternoon when we met for lunch at the Texas Roadhouse. Over the last few weeks, we've been growing closer, talking or texting, and meeting up whenever we can. And although we haven't had any physical contact, what's happening between us feels corrupt. I can feel myself sliding down a slippery slope from attraction to a full-blown affair.

After we ate on Friday, Chris stood outside my Jeep smoking a cigarette while we said goodbye.

"I'll text you later," I said.

"Not if I text you first," he said. This is our version of the old "you hang up first, no, you hang up first" telephone game. We laughed.

"Can I kiss you?" he asked.

I was taken aback by his abrupt boldness. "No," I said, wondering if he was joking.

"Please?"

"No," I said again, smiling, because then I knew he was serious. "I have to go," I said as I pushed the window button and shifted into drive.

I could see him in my rearview mirror, watching me drive away, cigarette in one hand, the other in his sweatshirt pocket. I thought about turning around to tell him I'd changed my mind. But I hadn't.

I haven't. The thought alone feels wrong. We're both married to other people. And regardless of the problems between Ronnie and me, he doesn't deserve that. His love should be enough for me. I'm also not a cheater, and I don't mess around with men who are taken. I tried to put it out of my mind.

But Sunday, as Ronnie drove us to Amherst to see Alita at college, Chris's words kept playing in my mind. *Can I kiss you?* I watched out the window, daydreaming about him, as the greens, whites, and pinks passed by in a blur and Serena slept in the back seat.

When my phone dinged, I held my breath and glanced at Ronnie. His eyes stayed on the road ahead. I pulled my iPhone from my purse and turned it toward the passenger window, away from him. My heart raced when I saw Chris's name.

Hi, was all he said.

I responded quickly. *Hi.*

"What time do you think we'll get there?" I asked Ronnie to distract him from what I was doing.

"How do I know?" he said.

His dismissive response only reminded me why talking to Chris felt so good.

For the next hour, while Serena slept, Chris and I went back and forth. He missed me. I missed him too. He couldn't wait to see me. I felt the same way.

I glanced at Ronnie to see if he noticed I wasn't really there. He didn't seem to; he trusted me completely.

He shouldn't have.

Chris and I met here tonight, at Gloucester's Trinity Church beginner's meeting, strictly for recovery-related purposes. That's what I told myself, anyway. But the meeting ended half an hour ago, and we've been sitting in his truck since. Ours are the only two vehicles left in the parking lot. Although Ronnie is expecting me, it's near impossible to pull myself away. Our conversation has taken on a life of its own. It's the first time we've talked at length about my past and my Aunt Julie.

"Other than Debbie, she was the only person who paid attention to me when I was a kid. Of course, she was crazy," I say, letting out a short laugh. I know it's not funny, but this is what I do when I get nervous.

Chris reaches over and puts his hand on mine. When I glance at him, I can see the sadness in his eyes, and I feel bad for causing it. Hearing these things must be difficult, since he knew me back then. I wonder if he feels like he should've done something to help me. Of course he had no idea what was going on—the only people who did know were involved, and they weren't talking about it. And even if Chris had known, it's not like he could've done anything. He was just a kid too.

As much as I want to tell him everything, I'm still not sure I should. I'm not only worried about his feelings, I'm also anxious about how he'll take the news, and whether he'll think less of me. The woman he sees today—the strong, seemingly confident attorney—is a far cry from who I used to be and the person I still greatly resemble on the inside.

Regardless of what might happen or what he'll think, this is something I have to do. I have to be honest about who I am and where I've been. I look down at my lap and continue. "My mother was getting high, Walter was drunk most of the time, and all they did was fight whenever they were home at the same time. I wanted to get away, and Aunt Julie was there to help me do that."

I pause, gathering courage to tell him about what happens next.

"She had friends who had pot and pills, and guys who liked young girls. They were more than happy to give me drugs and money for... things. Sexual things. Almost all of the women I knew, including my mother, were doing the same thing, so it seemed normal even though I had a feeling it wasn't. And, of course, it made me feel shitty about myself."

I glance at him just long enough to see that his eyes are moist. I wonder what he's thinking, what *I* would think hearing these things. After all these years, I can still hear that voice telling me I'm worthless and dirty. Is it possible that he hears it too?

The pressure building in my chest has worked its way up into my throat where it sits like a boulder. I'll cry if I don't stop it. I take a deep breath and push it back down. His light touch on my hand tells me it's safe to continue.

"It went on for a few years. At one point, the police even became involved. They interrogated me when I was thirteen and covered with poison ivy that had nearly swollen my right eye shut. It was just two detectives, my mother and me in one of their shoebox offices; two men, a woman, and a child. No lawyer. They knew exactly what they were doing."

"That's fucked up," he says.

"Sure was."

"All of it, I mean."

"Yeah, I know," I say, looking away.

"I can't believe all that was going on. I had no idea that stuff like that even happened in Gloucester."

"Well, it's not like anybody was out screaming it from the rooftops," I say, and chuckle again, this time without smiling.

"I'm so sorry you had to grow up that way." I can feel his eyes on me, but I can't look at him. His soothing tone and words dripping with compassion are what break me. This is what I've always wanted, for somebody to know the truth and accept me anyway.

We sit in silence for a few minutes. He's giving me time to gather myself; I can sense he knows what I need.

This time when I look at him, he's crying—full-blown snot and tears. His visible pain makes me look away again, and I have no doubt that if he could go back and change things for me he would.

The intimacy of this moment makes me think of what's missing elsewhere. Ronnie's face drifts through my mind. The man I share every day with, my husband of seven years, doesn't know any of these things about me. It's not necessarily his fault; I've never given him the option to show me whether he can handle the weight of my past. Although he's never asked. Having deep conversations about the intimate details of our lives isn't something we do. I don't trust him to look beyond who I was, who I really am.

But Chris is different. He knew me back then, and he wants to know more.

"Did your Aunt Julie ever get in trouble?"

I wipe my eyes and tuck my hair behind my ear, grateful for an easy, factual question. "Not that I know of. She didn't go to jail or anything. They might have questioned her, but I don't know. I ran away to Texas the day after I went to the police station, and when I got back, there was a social worker waiting at the airport to take me to my first foster home. I never heard another thing about it."

"Holy shit, Gail. I'm blown away by how remarkable you are."

I look at him briefly, my head tilted to the left and my eyebrows drawn together, and then look away toward the dilapidated wall beyond the windshield. I'm sure he recognizes the disbelief in my expression. Of all the words I would use to describe myself, "remarkable" isn't one of them. It's not that

I don't see the good qualities I possess, but those pale in comparison to all that is wrong with me.

"I mean it," he says. Hearing the sincerity in his voice, I turn to face him again. This time, I don't look away. My hand feels cool and light when he lifts his away and reaches for my face. He cups my chin and locks his eyes on mine. "Seriously. I've never felt more love for anybody than I do for you in this moment." The look in his eyes makes me feel supported, like he wants to join me in my deepest, darkest places.

"Can I kiss you?"

"Yes," I say before he leans in. As his lips touch mine, I become acutely aware of my entire body. It feels alive and present—the blood rushing through my veins and every hair standing on end.

"Oh my God," I say, looking away from him.

"Yeah," he says.

I turn back to him. "I really have to go."

"Okay," he says, as he brushes the back of his hand along the curve of my cheek. "Thank you."

19

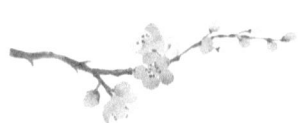

RUNAWAY TRAIN

I hear Ronnie coming down the stairs just before I see him standing in the kitchen doorway. He must've heard me come in a few minutes ago. I'm at the peninsula thumbing through the day's stack of mail when he speaks.

"Why are you so late?"

"I'm not. The meeting got over at eight."

"Yeah, okay," he says, his nostrils flaring. He comes further into the kitchen, then turns and walks back toward the doorway, pacing like a caged animal. My neck muscles tighten.

"And why the fuck are you dressed like that to go to a meeting?" he asks as he waves his arm in my direction. I don't budge. I'm not worried he'll hurt me. Although he's got an angry disposition, he's never been violent with me.

"Dressed like what?" I look down at my black, spaghetti-strap camisole. "Oh. I didn't come home after court," I say with a slight nod toward where my jacket is hung on the back of a kitchen chair. "I was wearing my suit jacket."

"You're a liar," he says, his face red.

I am a liar, but I'm not lying about that.

"Look, Ronnie, it's right there."

"You're fucking around," he says.

Of course, he's not wrong. In the last two months, although Chris and I haven't gone all the way, we've come close. I want to be with him more than anything, and he wants to be with me.

"What are you talking about? I just went to a mee...." He cuts me off.

"You wouldn't go to a meeting dressed like a whore!" I look away, his words knocking the wind out of me like a punch in the stomach. He doesn't know that of all the words he could have chosen, that particular one brings back every shameful memory I've tried to bury.

I steel myself and take in a sharp breath before responding. "Ronnie, you need to keep your voice down. You're going to wake Serena."

"I don't give a shit," he says. "You're a fucking liar." With his last word, he lunges forward, picks up a counter stool, and throws it against the wall.

The crash makes me jump, but I stay rooted in place, frozen with the same fear I felt as a kid whenever a fight would break out in our apartment or when my mother's boyfriend, Walter, was having an angry-drunk instead of a happy one.

But this is different. Ronnie is *sober*, and in the nine years we've been together, aside from the one time he repeatedly slammed the portable crib onto the kitchen linoleum when it wouldn't collapse, I've never seen him so angry. I've told people that his bark is worse than his bite, but at the moment, I'm not so sure. One thing I do know is to keep my cool—something I learned from watching my mother talk Walter down. I also know better than to let anybody see when I'm afraid.

I steal a quick glance at the stool, and then back at Ronnie, where I lock my gaze as I listen for Serena above us. It's so quiet, I'd think I imagined the whole thing if the stool wasn't still lying sideways on the floor.

"You need to leave," I say, my tone clear and even, despite my shaking insides.

Ronnie walks to the stool, rights it, and then stands behind it, across the counter from me.

"I'm sorry, I didn't mean to do that." His voice is quiet now, his eyes are filled with tears and unmistakable pain.

It's my fault, I know. I'm sorry too, but I don't say that.

As much as I wish we didn't end up here, there's nothing I can do. There is no other choice to be made. Just like I was when it came to my mother and her drugs, and later with my own, I'm a passenger on a runaway train. I'm already gone.

20

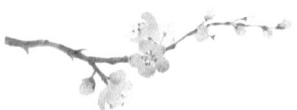

RESTRAINT

"**A**ttorney Nastasia," the court officer says, smiling as he greets me inside the front door of the courthouse, as he does just about every day. He doesn't know that today, I'm not here as an attorney—I'm here for a restraining order. But how could he know? I'm looking as respectable as ever in my fitted, navy blue suit.

"Good morning." I say, smiling back, cool and seemingly unflappable. I'm good at pretending, but my stomach and chest are tight with stress.

As I continue past the metal detectors and into the civil clerk's office, I feel like I'm having an out-of-body experience. Everything looks strange from this civilian perspective.

Relief overcomes me when I see that I don't know the woman behind the counter and she doesn't know me. It makes sense, because I never do civil work, but I was still worried about having to answer questions. For the moment at least, I can relax. She hands me a stack of forms to fill out.

When I'm done with the paperwork, I pass it back to the woman and stand off to the side to wait. With anything court-related, there's always a wait.

My thoughts are already consumed with having to go before a judge. The days of fearing those powerful black-robed judges are behind me, but this situation is different. I have to appear before a judge I know—someone who has presided over several of my criminal cases. I'll have to tell them, my colleagues, the courtroom staff, and whoever's in the audience what happened when Ronnie came downstairs last night.

My current dirty laundry is about to be aired for all to hear. I would have gone to any other courthouse if it were an option, but this is my district. The phrase "don't shit where you eat" keeps running through my head.

The only upside is that for this initial hearing, Ronnie won't be here. This part, the preliminary phase, is *ex parte*, legalese for "one-sided." It's like a warm-up, a way for me to ease into the shitshow that's coming. Soon, Ronnie will be served, and everything is going to change. I wish I didn't have to do it, but regardless of Ronnie's remorse about the way he acted last night, he's angry, and I can't take the chance it could happen again. The last thing I want is for Serena to feel the same fear I did as a kid. I also know he won't let me go if given the option. And I'm done.

"Your case will be called in session four," the clerk says as she slides my copy of the paperwork across the counter. I don't tell her I already know that. I've been practicing law in this building, and in that particular session, for over a year.

I press the elevator's call button like it's any other day. After a small group piles in, I move closer to the door so I can get out quickly.

My mind races as I step out onto the third floor where an anxious energy flows through the large, open space. There are people everywhere, some seated on wooden benches, others, including uniformed police officers who are standing together in conversation. Many of the faces are familiar; some I even consider friends. I nod and smile as I pass them on my way to the courtroom.

The clickity clack of my heels on the tile floor remind me of who I'm supposed to be when I'm here: a professional woman doing her job. Here, I rarely let anyone into my inner circle or share my personal business.

There was only one time I told a colleague about my past, and that was completely unplanned. I was in a smaller court back then, and I'd been practicing for less than a year. My client had gotten high, in violation of his probation contract, and Chet, his probation officer, wanted him to go to jail. Chet and I sat together while waiting for the case to be called.

"I'll never understand these people," Chet said.

"Yeah, it's hard to grasp if you're not an addict."

"Seriously, though, if you know that getting high will land you in jail, and you get high anyway, you're just an idiot."

I bit my lower lip, thinking I should just let it go. Of course, I couldn't.

"That's not true. Some of the smartest people I know have been addicts," I said, thinking of my mother.

"I don't agree," he said, his opinion firm.

"Well, I couldn't stop no matter what the consequences."

"Stop what?" he asked, his eyes wide as though he was about to hear some scandalous gossip.

"Fentanyl. Whatever I could get my hands on," I said, looking him in the eye. The truth exploded out of me like boiling milk spilling over the sides of a pot. As careful as I'd been to keep that part of my life hidden from people like him, I couldn't stop myself.

"Holy shit. Really?"

"Yes. I have a pretty shady past. But here I am. And it's been five years."

But that was then. It was my choice to share what I had with Chet. Today is different—I'm not in charge of who hears what.

It's a little before nine when I walk into the courtroom, and the audience is already full. I walk past them, through the swinging wooden gate, and take a seat where the lawyers sit. After a deep breath, I turn to look toward the galley and silently thank the universe that my calendar was empty today. I don't know how I'd handle being a lawyer and plaintiff on the same day.

As the other attorneys file in, I say hello and pretend everything is normal.

"Who's on the bench?" one of them asks.

"Are the custodies in yet?" asks another.

I can't answer their questions, but I'm glad that as far as they're concerned, it's business as usual. Best-case scenario at this point is they'll all be gone by the time I hear my name called.

Fifteen minutes later, the clerk waves me up to her desk. She waits until I'm standing directly in front of her before she leans forward and whispers: "Your case will be called in session six as soon as the judge can do it."

"Thank you," I say, holding back unexpected tears of relief and gratitude for her consideration for my privacy. The other session is much smaller than this one.

There are a handful of people in session six, a room about the size of my living room. Just as I had in the other courtroom, I walk through the wooden gate and sit with the other lawyers, still not sure of the protocol under the circumstances.

The cases are called, one by one, until all are resolved but mine, and the judge walks off the bench. "Could you close the session now?" the clerk asks the court officer. He gets up and locks the door. I'm confused. They don't usually lock up until all the work is done.

A few minutes later, the judge returns to the bench, and the clerk calls my case. That's when I realize they closed the session for me. The evidence of their compassion hits me like an unexpected wave breaking against my back. I inhale quickly in a desperate attempt to close the small crack that threatens to break me wide open.

"Good morning, Attorney Nastasia," the judge says. My tears come despite my attempt to stop them. Just a few minutes ago I seemed to have it all together and now I can barely speak. I try to respond, but that only makes it worse. I'm embarrassed, ashamed, and I'm worried that my mess, those parts of me I have so successfully contained, will come pouring out of me and into this part of my life. The judge is patient; he pauses to give me a moment to pull myself together. Although the way he's looking at me, like he wishes he could give me a hug, doesn't help.

Twenty minutes later, I've been granted a temporary restraining order. Ronnie has to stay away from me and our house. We'll have a full hearing next week, and after that, I'll be able to start over again.

21

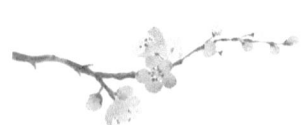

WHAT COMES NEXT

It's easy to think about what comes next on a rare weekday afternoon like this one, when the kids are at school, Chris has taken the day off from work, and I don't have to be in court. Even though it's the middle of the day, we're lying in bed together. It feels so good being here like this, I can almost forget about the bills, the judgment, and all the pain I've caused.

Now that there's a restraining order in effect, and Ronnie can't come within a hundred feet of our house, it's just me and the kids. But even though Jack and Serena are still with me, most days I feel as alone as I ever have. It's not just that I'm the only adult in the house; I also feel like I've lost all my friends. *Our* friends. They're on Ronnie's side. Not that I blame them—I am the one who's fallen in love with somebody else. But it still hurts.

That's not the only change. My meetings have been limited too, since I now have to depend solely on Jack to watch Serena, and babysitting his little sister is the last thing a recent high school graduate wants to do. He doesn't complain, which makes me feel guilty. I think he wants to please me the same way I wanted to please my mother.

I've also had to find new meetings. Ronnie and I went to many of the same ones, and considering I'm the one who ultimately chose to end our marriage, I should be the one to make changes. He would've stayed with me no matter what, I'm sure. So he can have the mutual meetings and friends. I'd rather avoid all those who've turned on me anyway.

On top of feeling disconnected from nearly all I've known for the last nine years, taking care of the house is more overwhelming than I could've imagined. Everything is on me—right down to taking out the trash. I'm also responsible for all the bills, and with Ronnie refusing to contribute anything, I'm drowning in expenses that used to be shared between us. I work as much as I can, but I still can't keep up. Not to mention, I'm exhausted all the time.

It's okay though, I can see the truth now. It wasn't the outside stuff I needed to be happy—the career, the marriage, the friends. It was this deep connection, this all-encompassing love I have with Chris.

In this moment, being with him is all that matters. His body belongs next to mine.

"I wish I could just crawl up inside you," he says. I wish he could too. That way, I'd never have to be without him.

"Me too," I say, rubbing my feet against his.

"We fit perfectly together," he says.

"I know. This is what I always thought love was supposed to feel like."

It's only been five months since I opened that first message from Chris. A little less than a month since Ronnie's been gone. Everything has been moving so fast. *Too fast*, I think some days. I had wanted to ease Serena into this monumental change, but she's with me most of the time, so I wasn't able to keep Chris a secret from her. She doesn't seem to mind him being around, especially since his daughter is just a year younger than her and they get along so well. I can only hope it isn't too much for her to handle.

"You need to get divorced, so we can start planning our future," I say, draping my leg over his. We both need to be free and clear of our other relationships before we can move forward. I filed my divorce paperwork a few weeks ago, and although he's told me his marriage was already on the verge of collapse before we met, he hasn't started his. I try not to think about it, but we're not any closer to our together-future than we were three months ago. I'm here in my house, and he's still living with his parents.

"I know, baby girl. I want to. I just don't have the money." I'm sure he's telling me the truth. His drug use put him in such a bad financial position he's having to shut down his business. He'll file as soon as he can. I'm sure he wants this as much as I do.

Although I still have questions about whether he's really clean. He says he is, but his pupils usually look like the tiny specks mine used to. If he's not, that's okay. For now anyway. I'll stand by him while he recovers. He needs me. And I've already given up so much to be with him.

"I can't wait to wake up next to the love of my life every morning," Chris says, pulling me closer

"Someday soon," I say. "We're meant to be."

"I want yours to be the last face I see before I die. My first, last, and always," he whispers in my ear. I love when he says that. His words remind me of our history, how we were together when we were twelve, and how we've come back together after all these years. It's destiny.

Back when we were just kids, I had no idea who I was or what I wanted. But now I'm an adult, and this is the feeling I've been searching for my whole life. As long as we can be together in the end, I'm willing to do whatever it takes.

I close my eyes and sink into the warmth of his body. Finally, everything makes sense. First, last, and always.

22

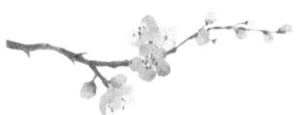

LITTLE GAIL

The loud "ding" of Chris's cell phone makes me jump. I look to where it's lying face down on my kitchen peninsula. I want to see if the message is from a woman—his soon-to-be-ex-wife, his ex-girlfriend Karen whom he reunited with around the same time we did, or somebody new.

But it isn't as simple as merely walking by for an accidental glimpse of the screen. I'll have to physically pick it up and turn it over, which would clearly be a boundary violation.

As I consider my options about whether to read Chris's text, I make my way to the other side of the counter closest to the phone. We've been fighting about this exact thing—trust and boundaries. The trust issue is mine.

I stopped trusting Chris when he moved into his apartment in Haverhill, a twenty-minute drive from me. At first, I'd been overjoyed. The place looked like something out of a movie with its brick walls and exposed ductwork. His willingness to live independently for the first time felt like proof of his desire to make our relationship work.

But two months later, shortly before he had to move, the apartment reeked of isolation and stale nicotine. The once pristine rooms resembled those I'd lived in as a child—flat surfaces covered with papers, empty cigarette packs, and half-filled coffee mugs. A rumpled blanket and pillow on the futon told me he'd been sleeping in the living room. I knew what it all meant. Just as I'd always known when my mother had relapsed, he was getting high for sure.

He was also talking to other women. That's where the boundary issue came from. Chris began demanding boundaries when I started looking at his phone. I'd also confronted him about an email to another woman I'd found on his open laptop. *"I'm sorry for leaving the way I did. I didn't know how to handle what was happening between us,"* it said. It sounded like an apology, but it felt like another reconnection. It made me wonder if I was just one of several past relationships he'd been looking to rekindle.

But that was six months ago. And on a Saturday like today, when Chris is here with his kids, all the fighting seems far away. Everything is right with the world.

Well, it was, anyway. Until I heard that notification sound. By the time his phone is within reach, I've made my decision. I flip it over.

It was great to see you too!... Let's go for a walk next weekend.

I hold my breath and look to the name at the top of the screen—Karen. My heart starts to pound as fast as it does when I step off the treadmill. He must've texted her first, saying it was great to see her. And it's news to me that they've been hanging around together. He should have told me that. If I was spending time with an ex-boyfriend, he'd certainly want to know.

I start to scroll up, but then I hear the bathroom doorknob turn. I quickly replace the phone and rush past the bathroom door to the living room. There, I stand at the glass door, pretending to look out at the wetlands beyond the backyard.

"Hey," Chris says from the dining room. "Where'd my baby go?" His voice sounds like music to me. Even at this moment, I love the song he sings.

"I'm in here."

"There she is," he says, smiling, as he rounds the corner. He comes up behind me, and puts his hands on my waist, his head on my shoulder.

"What are we looking at?"

"Nothing, just thinking," I say. I'm trying to keep my cool, to pretend the text doesn't matter. If I believe he loves me as much as he says, it shouldn't matter. I should trust him as much as I trusted Ronnie. Then again, Ronnie didn't talk to his exes, not once. And Chris lied to me. Again. As much as I'd like to stop being jealous and insecure, the feelings are so much bigger than me. It feels like the ground is moving under my feet.

"About?" he asks, nuzzling his face against my neck.

"You saw Karen?"

He pulls away immediately. Already missing the warmth of his body next to mine, I regret saying anything.

"What are you talking about?"

"She texted while you were in the bathroom. About seeing you."

"You looked at my phone?"

I turn to face him, but he's already walking in the direction of the kitchen, and the exit.

I follow him—the conversation isn't over. I also might need to try and stop him from leaving. "I couldn't help it," I say. "Are you going to answer me?"

He picks up his phone and looks at the text. I'm sure he wants to see exactly what it says so he doesn't give me more information than I already have. "Answer you about what?"

"It wasn't a big deal," he says as he tucks the phone in his sweatshirt pocket. "I told you, we're friends. And this is bullshit." He's getting ready to leave.

"What are you doing?"

"Leaving. Come on, kids. Time to go," he says as he walks toward the door. Both of his kids rush out behind him, stopping briefly inside the front door to put on their sneakers.

"Wait." I follow them.

"You're crazy," he says before walking out the door.

Maybe he's right. I can't stop myself from following him. I stand on the stoop and watch the three of them get in his truck. He lights a cigarette and turns on the ignition. He's still close enough that with the windows down, I can smell the smoke and hear music coming from his speakers.

A renewed sense of panic rises in me as he backs out of the driveway and pulls out onto the street. I recognize the feeling at once as Little Gail, the little girl whose father walked out on her when she was too young to remember him being there. She's always there, just below the surface, waiting to be loved without the fear of being left behind.

The kids wave goodbye, and I wave back. Chris doesn't turn to look at me. There's an ache in my chest, and my throat feels like it's closing. My mind races for something, anything that will make him turn around.

"If you leave, don't bother coming back," I yell, but I know I don't mean it. And I have no idea what I'll do if he does as I say.

23

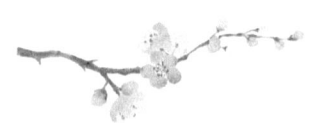

MORPHINE SULFATE

I'd just rounded the corner from the foyer into the kitchen when I saw something on the floor. My body responded, heart pounding, before I even had time to think. It looked like a pill.

Please let me be wrong. My first thought was more like a silent request to the universe. Chris had spent the weekend and at eight months into our relationship, I knew he was still struggling to stay clean.

It was the last thing I wanted to deal with today. After arguing nearly every case at court, my only desire was to come home to a quiet house, change out of my suit, into something comfy, and relax with mindless television for a while.

And, until a few minutes before I walked into the kitchen, everything seemed to be going as planned. Jack was out, and I had a couple hours to myself before I had to pick up Serena. Even Daisy, our ten-year-old cat, was outside. But now I was looking at something resembling a tablet even from several feet away.

A few more steps into the room confirmed what I already knew in my gut. I was right. It was a pill, and it had to be Chris's. I wasn't taking anything, and it certainly didn't belong to Serena or Jack.

I stood there for a full minute before launching into my investigation. Despite my curiosity, I wasn't sure I wanted to know the truth. Although I already did know. I've known all along. But just as I always did with my mother, I ignored the signs.

For a moment, I wished I was still in court, feeling respected and needed, doing good work and helping people. Lately, it's been the only thing keeping me from my relationship insanity—the same obsession I once had with drugs is now reserved for Chris.

When I picked it up and read the imprint, M 30, I was somewhat relieved by its unfamiliarity. I'd recognize a good pill for sure, the kind an addict would use to get high. Then again, in the seven years since I used any pills, something new could've come on the market. As much as I hated to admit it, I didn't know everything.

I considered getting rid of the pill, throwing it in the trash as though I hadn't seen it to begin with, but I needed to know what it was.

With my laptop already set up and open on the living room desk, I typed "pill identifier" into the search bar and waited.

Now, I have my answer. Morphine Sulfate. Fuck. Thirty milligrams. A high dosage. Chris isn't just dabbling—he's strung out. I roll the pill between my thumb and forefinger as I refresh the page. Of course, the results haven't changed. The truth is in my hand.

My first instinct is to text Chris, to tell him I know what he's been doing. I won't mention my find right away; instead, I'll let him squirm, wondering how I know. Then, like a witness identifying the defendant in a courtroom, I'll hurl the proof at him.

No, I can't do that. Even though the last year has been filled with pain and heartache, that's not the way I want our relationship to be. I don't want him to feel like he's on the stand with me. Besides, he'll just say it isn't his.

I've also been trying not to text him. I'm waiting for him to reach out first. He owes me an apology in a big way, and it doesn't seem like he's planning on paying up anytime soon. It's already been over twenty-four hours since our last communication, when he said something almost unforgivable.

We were on the phone yesterday when I couldn't help but ask, yet again, if he'd filed his divorce paperwork.

"No. I told you I don't have the money."

I wouldn't let it go.

"Fine," he said. "Do you want to know the truth?"

"Of course," I said, although his tone made me think I didn't.

"Okay. I told Beth not to divorce me. I said, 'No matter what I do or what I say, don't sign any paperwork.' I wanted to make sure I wouldn't do something stupid like marry you."

I stayed silent. I felt like I'd been punched in the stomach, the wind knocked out of me.

"Listen, Gail, we can't keep doing this. Maybe someday we'll be able to come back together when we're both in a different place, but this isn't working." Then he hung up.

His words hung in the air. He'd never said anything quite that mean. Maybe we really were coming to the end. The thought of him pulling away made me feel wobbly, like a top at the end of its spin.

But that was yesterday, and before finding the pill, even without an apology, I was just about ready to forgive him. He didn't mean what he'd said. We both say mean things when we get angry. That's how it is with us.

I could just tell him I found a pill on the floor. Be honest with him, unlike he's been with me.

But then what? There's a reason he keeps these things from me. He's not ready to stop. It's no different than when I would lie to Ronnie, when I'd take his pills and replace them with vitamin C so he wouldn't notice them missing. I hadn't wanted Ronnie to leave me anymore than Chris wants me to leave him.

This must be payback, the universe's way of leveling the playing field. With Ronnie, I'd been the sneaky addict. Now I get to be on the receiving end. But I've already done my time in that role. Hadn't growing up with an addict been enough?

I should just take it.

The thought surprises me. As much as I don't want to get high, it would definitely solve the I'm-clean-and-Chris-isn't problem. We'd be able to be together.

I bolt from the chair as though propelled by some unseen force and race to the closest bathroom, the offending pill in my hand.

But I hesitate when I get to the open toilet. What if Chris says I was lying, that I didn't find anything? It wouldn't be the first time. Did it really make sense to dispose of the evidence? I wouldn't be a very good lawyer if I didn't hang onto the proof.

Instead of flushing the pill, I carry it to the kitchen cabinet where all household medicines are kept and slip it into a bottle with leftover antibiotics.

With my exhibit safe, I can focus on how to approach Chris. I go back upstairs to my bedroom to think. I should call and tell him he's ruining my life.

But that's not true. This is all on me.

As much as I say I don't like the drama and want to have a normal life, I willingly stay in the cycle. I'm far from a victim—I'm a full-fledged volunteer if there ever was one, and I wouldn't know normal if it jumped up and bit off my nose. Never have and probably never will.

I'm pacing with the phone in my hand, when I press his name.

Chris picks up on the second ring. "Hey," he says.

"What's up?" I ask, my voice laced with hostility.

"What's wrong?"

He can tell there's something new, something beyond yesterday's conflict.

"I found a pill on the kitchen floor," I blurt.

"Okay. So?"

"So I looked it up."

"And?"

"And it's morphine," I say it slowly, like I'm talking to a child, getting more pissed by the second that he's making me work for a confession.

"Oh. It must've fallen out of my bag." At least he doesn't deny it's his. At least.

He sounds exactly like I would have seven years ago if Ronnie had found one of my pills on the floor, although that wouldn't have happened—I never lost or misplaced a painkiller. Still, calling Chris a liar right now will only make matters worse. I decide to let it go for the moment. "Okay," I say. "We'll talk about it later."

After I hang up, the house feels impossibly quiet. If I didn't know better, I'd swear that in the silence I can hear the pill calling my name.

I go back downstairs and again open the orange container. As I pour the contents into my palm and look for the offending pill, I find myself humming the Sesame Street song "One of These Things," where the kids pick which item in a group is different from the others.

It doesn't make sense that this tiny thing, the same chalky tablet that sent me into a panic less than an hour ago, is making me want to sing, but that is the nature of this beast. I know it as well as I know the color of my own eyes.

With the pill back in my hand, I notice how smooth it is. It would be so easy to just toss it down my throat. Just one. What harm can one do?

If I just lick it—

My feet respond to this unwelcome thought. They move toward the bathroom more quickly than my mind can catch up. The lid is still open, and before I can think any more about it, I toss the pill into the water and flush.

I watch as the swirling water takes the painkiller down into the darkness. Standing here, I half expect the drug to reappear and test me as if it knows I'm waiting, just as Chris does. Of course, it doesn't. And as much as I already miss having it as an option, I know I made the right choice in letting it go.

Chris, though, he's another story.

2010-2011

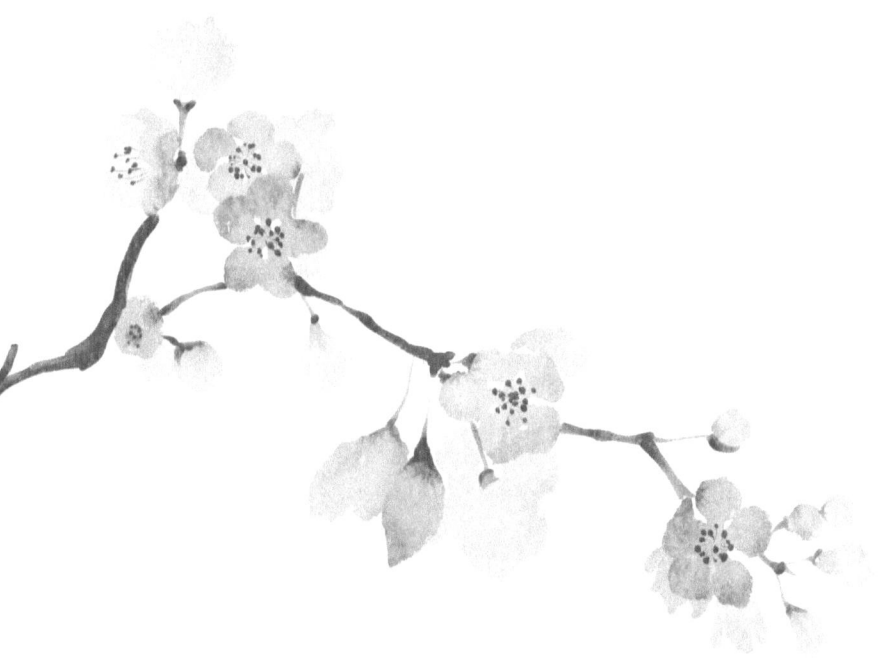

24

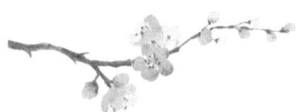

BLOCKED

Despite the frigid January air, I put the front windows of my Jeep halfway down and blast Gary Wright's "Love Is Alive" as I speed down I-90. I play the song twice, belting out the words while ignoring the tickle in my throat and letting my tears flow.

When it's done, I put the windows back up, turn the dial to soft rock, and wipe my face. "Fuck him." But it doesn't matter that I said the words out loud. I still don't mean them when it comes to Chris any more than I did when I said them about Percocet.

I pick up the phone to text him again, even though I know he won't respond. He should be with me this weekend. He's supposed to be. The tickets to *Rock of Ages* on Broadway were a Christmas present for him. And just like the trip to NYC I gave Ronnie for Christmas last year, it's one I couldn't really afford. In order to get them, I had to put off making my car payment. That's nothing new, I've been struggling with how to handle money my whole life. Only lately have I started really thinking about it as a relationship I need to foster—in the future.

At the moment, I can only think of Chris, who isn't here for what was supposed to be a romantic getaway. My daughter Alita is coming instead. I'm picking her up in western Massachusetts on my way to Manhattan.

I look down at my phone where my text hangs, undelivered. He's got my number blocked. Being ignored like this feels heavy; the weight of it sits in my belly like a stone, threatening to rise up into my chest and throat if I let it. When I click on the little telephone symbol, I hear Chris's voice telling me to leave a message. I don't. Even if he were to listen to it, he wouldn't call me back.

I step hard on the gas and swerve around an SUV that's driving too slowly for the fast lane. The driver gives me the finger, and I give it right back.

By the time I arrive at Alita's, I've managed to calm myself. I'm determined to make the best of this time with my daughter.

Alita comes right out when I honk my horn.

As she walks toward me, I see myself in her. We're the same height, and her face is shaped like mine. And now that my hair is back to its natural brown, and hers is shoulder-length, we look more alike than ever.

She smiles as she slides into the passenger's seat.

"Hi," I say as I lean in for a hug. "I'm glad you're coming with me. We haven't spent much time together lately."

"Me too," she says, as I pull away from the curb.

I'm trying to switch gears and look at this situation as an opportunity to grow. Some mother-daughter time will certainly be good for us. We've never done anything like this before. I can give her all of me for a couple of days, at least. I haven't been the best mother, but I'm here now. I want to do better. After nearly eight years of sobriety, it's about time.

"What's new?" I ask, knowing it's the only way to keep myself from rambling about my current drama.

She responds right away, and tells me about a recent plumbing issue she's having in her shared apartment.

I can hear her voice, but I'm not really listening. My thoughts are on my phone, which is facing down beside me on the console. All I want to do is pick it up and try to text Chris again. He's probably with Karen, and I bet they're talking about me. She hates me.

"Mom," Alita says, snapping me out of my mental tirade. "Are you listening?"

I'm guessing she's well-aware of my clear inability to talk about anything other than Chris.

"Yeah, I just have a lot on my mind." As I say it, I hear my mother's voice uttering the same words to me when I was fourteen. We'd been living in the apartment of her new boyfriend, Angel. They were fighting, and I was worried we'd have to leave.

"Are you going to break up?" I asked through the bathroom door.

"No," she said, as she passed me on her way to the bedroom she shared with him. I followed.

"He sounds pissed."

"Everything's fine, Gail. Don't worry about it." She stopped in front of the long dresser, picked up a brush and ran it through her hair.

"I am worried about it." When she didn't respond I asked: "Are you listening to me?"

"Sorry," she said, glancing at me. "I have a lot on my mind." Even back then I knew that heroin was all she could think about.

Alita stays quiet for a few minutes before speaking again. "So, what's going on with you and Chris?"

I'm so grateful she finally asked, that she's given me permission to let it all out. And I do. I tell her about his dishonesty, drug use, and the games he plays involving other women, even though I know I shouldn't be throwing all this nonsense at her. But she's twenty-one—an adult, I argue to myself. She feels more my equal, with us being just a little more than sixteen years apart. Still, I'm her mother. She should be the one talking, and I should be listening.

I glance over at her, and she nods as though in agreement with whatever I've just said. That's when I realize she's not looking at her cell phone like I would be. She's doing her best to engage. This is the only way she can be in my world.

Fifteen minutes pass before my phone vibrates. As I reach for it, I tell myself it's not him, so I don't get my hopes up.

"Mom, don't look at your phone while you're driving."

"I know, I'm sorry," I say, after looking at the screen and seeing it wasn't him. "I think I'm getting sick."

I toss the phone into the cup holder. My goal is to change the subject, but my throat really does hurt when I swallow. "I'm not feeling great," I add, realizing that's another mom-ism, a phrase she used often. Maybe she had a weak immune system, or maybe her body was reacting to the hell she put it through. Just like mine is now.

Alita and I sing along with the radio together for the remainder of the ride. It's easier for me than trying to engage. I imagine that's true for Alita too. I'm sure she doesn't want to hear about my love life, and we both love to sing.

By the time we arrive at the hotel, I'm clearing my throat often, and I've developed a cough. It's nothing major, just a slight irritation that I'm hoping will get better once I'm settled. A little rest can't hurt after such a long, emotionally draining day.

Our room is modern and clean. It's perfect. I put my bag on the bed closest to the window and pull the drapes back. The city view is stunning, but even as I look out at the tall buildings and matchbox-like yellow cabs, I'm still thinking about Chris.

You're here now. Put the guy aside. You can pick him back up tomorrow. Enjoy this. Spend some time with Alita. That's my plan, but first, I need a few minutes alone with my phone.

"I'm going to get cleaned up," I say, taking out my makeup pouch. It's my cover, although Alita, who's already on her bed with a book, probably wouldn't have noticed my absence.

Once the door is closed, I text: "Why are you ignoring me?!?!?" The emphasis is only meant for me, since I know I'm still blocked. Like the other eight messages before it, this one doesn't deliver.

I put the phone face down and sit on the closed toilet. Now that I'm alone, I can let myself cry again. The tears come quickly as though they've been pooling behind my eyes, waiting for me to give them permission to fall. I watch my reflection as I weep. It's ridiculous and pitiful. I'm not some teenage, lovesick kid. I'm a soon-to-be divorced mother of three, and practicing criminal defense attorney. I've been through so much worse. But we were supposed to be together forever. Boo hoo.

Five minutes; that's all the time I allow myself to wallow. I stand and take a deep breath. Then, I drench one of the crisp white facecloths in hot water and hold it close to my face. The steam momentarily subdues the cough that's triggered whenever I inhale.

The second time I wet the cloth, the water is ice cold. This time when I hold it to my skin, it sends an invigorating shiver through my body. I take a deep breath, look into my eyes, and whisper, "You can do this."

During the brisk walk to the theater, my cough is worse than ever. I blame the dry winter air. But now, even though I'm seated inside, it still won't stop.

"I'm sorry." I look at Alita who's sitting to my left, speaking loud enough so all those surrounding us can hear. It's embarrassing that I don't have control over my own body. I take a sip of my bottled water to try to suppress the scratch in my throat.

The show has only just begun when my hacking becomes so incessant, I'm sure ruining this experience for everybody within earshot. My body is like a three year old who knows it's quiet time. People are staring.

"I'll be back," I say, hoping movement will help. We're seated six rows from the nearest exit, and, gratefully, my seat is on the end.

I go to the back of the theater, but it doesn't do any good. Instead of slowing me down, the move has thrown me into a full-on coughing fit. People are turning in their seats, and flashing angry eyes my way. I'm torn. I don't know what to do. I have to get out of here, but I don't want to leave Alita alone. Obviously, she can take care of herself; not only is she on her own at college, she even managed to work out the financing by herself. My body makes the ultimate decision. It's calling the shots.

Leaving the theater, I hit the sidewalk in search of cough drops. I don't have to go far. There's a small convenience store just a few buildings down.

People gawk at me, the coughing lady, as I make my way back to the theater. The man at the door doesn't need to see my ticket since he recognizes me. During my short time in Manhattan's theater district, I've made quite an impression.

I'm still standing at the back of the room when the play ends. From the enthusiastic applause, I assume it was a hit. I missed so much of it, I can't even say what the show was about.

Alita meets me near the exit.

"Sorry, honey. I couldn't stop coughing."

"That's okay."

I want to tell her it's not okay, that this is my fault, and I've done this to myself. I could tell her I feel guilty and that this is not the way I wanted our night to go. But I'm sure she doesn't want to hear that either; I can't make this about me too. "What did you think of the play?" I ask instead.

"It was good. I liked it."

We walk to the hotel in silence, both of us shivering.

It's after eleven by the time we get back to our room, and even later when we slip into our beds, exhausted.

But the second I lie down my coughing starts up again. It's nonstop unless

I'm sitting up. Alita doesn't say anything, but I can hear her moving around. Now I'm keeping her awake. I prop myself up with pillows and try to sleep.

Finally, I find the sweet spot, and I'm just about to drift off when I realize there's another way for me to contact Chris—Skype. I can't believe I didn't think of it sooner. It's one of the ways we communicated when we were a secret. I know he wouldn't have thought to block me there. If he even uses it still.

I reach for my laptop on the nightstand, excited and hopeful.

Opening it, I dim the screen light as much as possible and type: "Are you there? Please answer me."

"Gail, you hung up on me," he responds right away. My first thought is whether his immediate response means he was already messaging with somebody (it wouldn't be the first time), but I put the thought out of my mind. It won't do me any good to go down that road, not right now.

The conversation goes on for two hours under my blanket while Alita asks me repeatedly to shut off the computer. We go over our usual arguments about trust, control, and boundaries before we're back together again. He loves me; I know he does. Beneath all the insanity of addiction, he will always choose me.

25

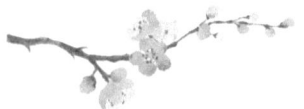

BREAKDOWN

Now that Alita is back at her place, I can relax. As much as I wanted to enjoy my time with her, I couldn't do anything other than obsess about Chris. I have to talk to him. I need to hear his voice and know that we're really okay.

As I pull away from the curb, I call him. It goes straight to voicemail.

I text him as I turn onto Route 202. It doesn't deliver. I feel the familiar ache in my stomach. Little Gail. I tap open the Skype app and message him. "Why am I still blocked?"

He responds a few minutes later. "I didn't say I was going to unblock you yet. We need to see how things go before I do that."

Fuck! I yell. *He's playing with me.* "Fuck this," I type and hit send before flinging my phone onto the passenger seat. When I turn my eyes back to the road, I see brake lights in front of me and they're coming up fast. I slam on my brakes and swerve to the right, just in time to avoid a collision. My heart pounds as traffic starts moving again.

I think about pulling over, but I just want to get home. Ronnie will be dropping Serena off soon after I get back, and I'm in no shape to parent a six-year-old. Who am I kidding? I'm in no shape to be a parent at all. I never have been. I don't know how to love and be loved. My head is spinning with negative thoughts; round and round they go like a scratched album skipping on a turntable.

I'm spiraling. I should pull over. But I can't stop. I need to get home. I have to keep moving and pay attention. No more texting and driving.

Tucking my hair behind my ear, I reach for the radio hoping music will help. I need some kind of relief.

The thought of getting high doesn't even cross my mind. After all the years I've been clean, I know well enough that any substance will only make things worse.

A cigarette, on the other hand, sounds like a good idea. It's been over seven years since I had one, but I still remember the immediate sense of peace I got from the first drag. But then, every puff after that made me want to quit. It was so hard to finally put them down for good. I know for a fact that one drag, the one that gives me a head rush, is all it'll take to turn me back into a full-fledged, pack-a-day smoker. Then, on top of being a failure at relationships, I'll again have the added shame of a nicotine addiction. That's the last thing I need.

But something has to give. Seven and a half years clean and sober, yet here I am, a complete basket case.

I'm in the far right lane when I notice the gully. There's no guardrail.

If I go fast enough and turn my wheel hard to the right...

The thought takes me by surprise. It's been years since I've felt like ending my life. But what else can I do? I have no idea how to live like a normal person, and I can't get high.

But you are getting high. I look to the passenger seat as though somebody else has spoken, but of course it's empty. The words came from inside of me.

I know the truth; I always have. Being with Chris feels as euphoric as fentanyl did at first, its warmth spreading through my body like hot tea on a cold night. But just as opiates turned on me, leaving me desperate when they were gone, Chris leaves me with the same pain of withdrawal.

You can't stay clean and live dirty. That's it. I get it now. The saying I've been hearing for years suddenly becomes clear. Sure, I've been clean, not using any drugs, but I'm living the same way I did when I was using. I haven't changed much at all.

I don't know what to do next.

"You could pray," I hear myself say out loud. *Yeah, that'll work,* my inner voice responds sarcastically. It's not the first time the idea has crossed my mind. Having been a member of twelve-step programs for the better part of my life, prayer has always been suggested by others. In the few times I've tried it over the years, I've been less than impressed with the results.

Although if I'm being honest, I'm willing to use all kinds of things to feel better. Prayer has always seemed like going one step too far. I'll reach for something that isn't good for me before turning to something I can't see or explain.

But the idea sounds much less ridiculous than it would have an hour ago. At the moment, I'm willing to try anything to make this ache go away.

I turn the radio off. I'm desperate enough to let there be silence.

"Listen," I say to the space around me, unsure of to what or whom I'm speaking. "I don't know what you want from me, but I'm still here, so I guess there must be something. Show me what I'm supposed to do."

The knot in my belly begins to loosen as I take a deep breath and blow it out. I pull a napkin from the console and wipe my face. My breathing slows.

For a moment, I just sit in the quiet, feeling a bit ridiculous.

Call Kate. That's my next thought. There's only one Kate in my life these days, and although she's not my sponsor, or even a really close friend, I do as the voice says.

I reach for my phone and dial Kate's number. She answers on the first ring. We talk for an hour. I tell her about what's happening with Chris, how I'm feeling, and that I know it's time for change. She listens.

By the time I pull into my driveway, my face is dry, and my eyes are clear. Nothing has changed with Chris. He probably still has me blocked, but I'm okay. There was no rainbow or burning bush along the way, but I made it home. I'm still alive.

26

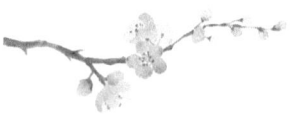

CRAZY

Less than half an hour ago, Chris and I were on our way to his parents' house. The warm summer air blew through my Jeep's open windows as we talked and laughed, enjoying each other's company. Everything felt perfect. We were like a normal couple going for a Saturday family visit. But I know better than to trust our brief interludes of peace.

Things took a turn for the worse when I heard the shrill notification sound of a Karen-text. Despite all that's happened between her and me, Chris still keeps her close.

Like Pavlov's dog, my body's typical response kicked into gear: a rush of gut-clenching anxiety followed by a wave of nausea.

Chris picked up his phone.

"What does she want?" I asked, my voice unfamiliarly high.

"Just saying hello."

"Why is she texting you today? She knows we're always together on Saturdays."

I could see from his expression that I should let it go, but I couldn't. I don't know how to let things go.

"I don't know. Why is it such a big deal?"

"I just don't understand why she's so important to you. You know how much she hates me."

"Listen, Gail, I'm not doing this shit with you. Not today."

We went back and forth a few more times, our typical argument where she's concerned. Then he slowed down, his eyes darting left and right, scanning the area.

"What are you doing?" I asked, knowing full well he was looking for a place to turn around.

"Going back to get my car."

The words hit me like a physical blow. My mind started racing with thoughts of him leaving and not coming back.

We both saw the turnaround shoulder at the same time. As he started to turn the wheel into it, I panicked.

"Chris, stop. Please. We have to be able to talk through these things and…" I reached over and grabbed the wheel. He held firm. We struggled over control. He pulled to the right as I pushed to the left to keep us on the road—to keep him with me. I couldn't stop myself. Even though I felt the insanity of the moment, I couldn't take my hands off the steering wheel. The thought of him leaving me was worse than the possibility of getting us both killed.

"What's wrong with you?" he asked, shifting his focus between me and the road, his brows drawn together, his eyes wild. He gripped the wheel with both hands and pulled hard to the right. "You're fucking crazy!" he yelled. As it slid from my grasp, I finally let go.

His words snapped me back into a state of reasonableness. I turned away so he wouldn't see the pain in my face. Maybe he was right. I've always questioned my sanity, especially since schizophrenia runs in my mother's side of the family. My grandmother, Aunt Julie, and Uncle Bobby had all spent time in the psych ward at some point. "If I go crazy, don't tell me," I've said to more than one boyfriend over the years, only half joking.

As I watch the landscape blur past through my tears, I keep hearing his words. I'm thinking about all that's happened over the last two years; the back and forth and the fighting. How last year, after I signed the house over to Ronnie in the divorce, Chris and I moved into an apartment together. I thought we'd go back to how we were in the beginning, and that he would again become my safe place. But he hasn't. Far from it.

Now, he sometimes lives with me, he sometimes doesn't, and I never know if he'll be at the apartment when I get home. My stomach muscles clench in anticipation whenever I turn onto my street, wondering whether I'll see Chris's car parked out front. I know my body is responding to issues from my past and not to whether Chris is there, but either way, I can't help it. A psychiatrist would probably say I'm suffering from Post-Traumatic

Stress Disorder related to my childhood, but Chris could be right; maybe I am crazy.

Or maybe his being back and forth isn't something I *should* accept. It's not normal. I'm thinking that anyone in my situation would respond the way I am. Well, maybe not quite as extreme. But if any "normal" person would have a negative reaction to being left, it makes sense that given my history, mine would be worse.

The more I think about it, the less crazy my behavior seems. After all, I never acted this way with Ronnie. Not once in our nine years together did I grab the steering wheel. I didn't go through his phone or feel the need to hunt him down. With him, I was calm, secure, and rational.

Ronnie showed up every day with a love that was steady and reliable. He didn't lie or play games. I never had to question whether his car would be in the driveway when I got home. Although he and I weren't meant for each other, he brought out the best in me.

Chris's love is the complete opposite. It's loud and dramatic. One minute, he makes me feel like I'm the only woman on the planet, and the next, like I'm completely worthless. It's the same kind of love I knew as a child—there one minute and gone the next. As a kid, I thought if I could just be better, quieter... less me, I wouldn't be left alone. I guess I still think the same way.

But my parents' failure to care for me had nothing to do with how I behaved. They weren't capable of being who I needed them to be. Neither is Chris.

I'm not crazy—I've just been doing the same thing over and over, expecting a different result. Okay, maybe I am a *little* crazy.

27

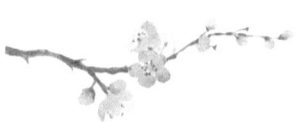

KARMA

When I left my apartment at two this morning, setting off in the dark for this journey to the airport, it had just started to snow. Now that I'm on the highway heading north, it looks like a blizzard. I can barely see ten feet ahead of me or go more than thirty miles per hour. And the wind is blowing so hard, my Jeep slides sideways every few feet. I can't help but think this must be karma for everything I've gotten wrong over this last year; the list is long. But I'm ready to put all that behind me. I'm on a spiritual quest.

The idea for the trip seemed to come about wholly by accident. One afternoon a few weeks ago, I'd been lying on my bed, staring at the ceiling, thinking about what to do next, when my eye was drawn to the bookcase. There, I spotted an orange-spined book, unlike all those surrounding it. I knew what it was—*A New Earth* by Eckhart Tolle. It didn't belong to me, and in the six months that it had been in my possession, not once had it ever occurred to me to read it.

Seeing the book got me thinking. Of all the things I'd tried to make change in my life, picking up a book about spirituality, something I thought of as "woo woo" and "out there," wasn't even on my list. The word alone—spirituality—made me flinch. Since returning from Manhattan, I'd been keeping up with the commitments I'd made to myself: praying every day, going to twelve-step meetings regularly, and meeting monthly with three other women in my living room.

Still, even with all the recovery work, I could hear that voice inside telling me I was worthless. I needed something more. That's what brought me to the bookcase. When I pulled the book from the shelf and saw chapter titles like "Breaking Free" and "Finding Who You Truly Are," it seemed necessary.

Since I had some time before having to pick Serena up from daycare, I lay back down and started to read from the beginning.

An hour later, I was a quarter of the way through. If I could've kept going, I would have. The pages were filled with insights I so desperately needed, and I was eager to learn more. Tolle's words had already shown me how my thoughts were most often in the past and future, not in the present moment. I understood completely why I'd been doing that—I thought if I could just figure out what had gone wrong in the past, I could do things differently. And only then could I imagine a better, more hopeful future.

Tolle's words reminded me of twelve-step sayings I'd grown up hearing: "If you have one foot in yesterday and one foot in tomorrow, you're pissing all over today" and "Keep your head where your feet are." His solution was the same: meditate. Stay present.

The concept was logical, of course. But for me, it felt impossible. How was I supposed to stop my thoughts from taking over? I'd tried meditating several times. My mind refused to rest in the present moment for more than a minute, if that, which made sense, because for me, the present was, and had always been, dark and painful—a place where I wouldn't want to visit, never mind live.

I needed to know more about meditation and Mr. Tolle. When I looked him up online that night, I saw that he was scheduled to appear in Vancouver a month later. I couldn't afford it any more than the other trips I'd taken, but I needed to see Tolle in person. I'd also never been to Canada or the west coast. Best of all, it gave me something healthy to obsess about.

My first inclination when planning the trip had been to include Chris. We would travel to Vancouver together in search of a solution to his addiction to pills and my addiction to him. It was a perfect chance for us to heal as a couple. He bought the airline tickets, and I paid for the event. I even called Karen and tried to make peace with her. We're still not friends; I don't trust her any more than I trust Chris, but at the time, it felt good to put the fighting behind us. For two weeks, Chris and I were the happy couple I knew we could be.

A few days before the trip, I found out Chris was using. The day after that, he bailed out of this trip just as he'd bailed out of Manhattan.

I considered canceling too. The thought of traveling to another country alone makes me sweat. But I can't forget why I wanted to come on this trip to begin with—to silence the voice that tells me I'm worthless. That voice is the reason I keep going back to Chris. It's quiet during the good times with him, because for those brief periods, I feel like I'm worth something.

But now I know Chris canceling was the best thing that could have happened. As anxious as I am to be driving in the snow and flying to a foreign land by myself, this feels like something I have to do. I refuse to believe I'm doomed to a life of constant heartache. This is my opportunity to find another way.

28

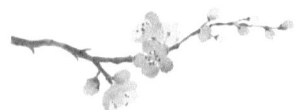

SHE IS NOT WORTH IT

Last weekend, despite his obvious distance in the months since Vancouver, Chris surprised me with a party for my birthday.

That Saturday started out as one of the best days we've ever had. His parents and sisters came to my house with a cake and gifts. They sang "Happy Birthday."

The only party I'd ever had before then was for my fourteenth birthday, when my mother, being in the throes of heroin addiction, bought a keg for me and my sister, who had turned sixteen five days before. Ronnie had always given me gifts, but parties weren't a thing, and I wasn't used to being celebrated.

But when Chris's family left us alone, he said he had to go. There was no changing his mind. He texted later that night, but I've hardly seen him in a week. This is the longest he and I have gone without seeing each other since we stopped sneaking around.

Today, we finally had plans to talk. I've been waiting all day for him to come over, with the sound turned up on my phone for fear I'll miss his text. Even so, I've looked at my phone every ten minutes. He's texted a few times throughout the day to tell me he was on his way, but he's still not here and it's past eight.

Time is moving so slowly it feels like it's standing still. And I'm running out of things to do to occupy myself. If not for my new meditation practice, I'd be out of my mind. As it is, I can only manage five minutes of silence at a time, but it's a start. I just wish he would get here already.

After one last look out the window at the empty driveway, I sit on the edge of the bed and text him again.

Where are you?

A minute later, his response pops up. *I'm on my way.*

You've already said that. What's taking you so long?

The three dots appear, but then they're gone. I stare at my phone, waiting for more. Nothing. I wait. Five minutes… ten. Fifteen minutes have passed before the dots are there again. As I wait for his reply, I think about driving to Gloucester to hunt him down. It wouldn't be the first time. Hell, he wouldn't even be the first guy I've tracked. Once I get an idea in my head, I can't let it go. But Serena is asleep in her room.

Three dots again, and then—*I have to tell you something.*

I feel the familiar weight of panic on my chest. For all the times I've asked him to just be honest with me, right now I only want him to be here.

What is it? I type the words even though I don't want to hear it. I know it can't be good.

I'm going to send you something, but I have to email it. The file is too big to text.

Wtf, Chris. What is it?

You'll see.

A few minutes later, there's an email in my inbox. The subject line is empty. My heart races as I click to open it.

I'm sorry your dealing with this.. I really am

R u with gail?

I am not

Were u with her last night?

I was

Did u have sex?

Heavy petting. No intercourse

*Does **** know?*

She does not

Wait…who is dealing with what? And who is ****? After reading the first few lines, I realize this is a text-chat history, a conversation between Chris and Karen.

Karen. She's never very far away.

I've tried to get to know her better over the last few weeks. We've even talked on the phone a few times since that initial conversation. In fact, we talked last night. I told her I was with Chris. What I don't understand is why she's asking him if we had sex. What does she care? Why is he lying to her, and why would it matter whether the mystery person knows anything about what Chris and I do?

I should stop reading. I've been doing so much better lately with prayer, meditation, and I'm calling other women more often. Not only have I been obsessing less, I've also been more present for my kids and clients.

But I can't help but read on.

She is nuts....
She showed up at the shop last night.
Please…please..do not fuck it up with ****....for her...she is not worth it
Look karen... **** has shown me what a normal healthy relationship
could look like again

The understanding that *she* is *me* hits me with the force of a wrecking ball. Chris is saying I am nuts, while Karen is telling him not to "fuck it up" with somebody else. This is his way of telling me what he's been doing behind my back.

Chris...why would u heavy pet with gail then....stop it!
She has made all the difference in the world as far as not walking right
back into the cycle of insanity
It was stupid and I will tell ****

I feel like I might be sick. I close my eyes and wait for the wave to pass. I wish I could stop here, knowing as much as I do—already too much. But that's not possible. I won't rest until I have all the facts. My need to examine and dissect every situation is insatiable.

"You can do this," I say aloud, before taking a deep breath. I open my eyes and finish reading what's left of the nearly two-page transcript of Karen text-lecturing Chris about how he needs to be honest with the woman behind the asterisks, and Chris telling Karen that the other woman should also be honest with her husband. *Her husband.* Surprise, surprise, the mystery woman is married too. Not so much a mystery now either, since Gloucester is a small town. I had my suspicions about who it could be. After looking at her Facebook, where we had once been friends, now there is no question—I've been unfriended.

I close my laptop and pick up my phone, ready to fire off a text to Chris, but then put it back down. Nothing good can come from a quick reaction. I need to think about this. After all, thinking is what I do best.

She is not worth it. Karen's words ring in my head. In Chris's response, while not directly saying so, he seemed to agree with her. He said it was stupid to be with me when he had this other person waiting for him. Not that he told her the whole truth. In the true story, we'd gone to a restaurant for dinner, and then to his shop where we talked. Then we made love. Before leaving, we decided together to put the past behind us and that we were the real deal.

I pick up my phone and type: *If you wanted us to be over, all you had to do was say so.* I block his number. As much as I want to hear his response, it's clear that this love, or whatever it is, will only continue to cause me pain. Our relationship is over. It has to be.

But even as I set the phone down, my thumb hovers over the settings. The silence feels wrong. What if he's trying to reach me? What if he has an explanation?

An hour later, I unblock him. Half an hour after that, I'm lying in bed with my head propped against the headboard, and Chris and I are texting back and forth. He has a lot to say.

I'm sorry. So, so sorry. I screwed up. Being with her was a mistake. That's why I sent you the whole chat, so you'd know everything. You deserve complete honesty from me. It's time I gave you that. You're who I want to be with. You and only you BBG. I'll make it up to you, I promise.

It's past midnight by the time I put my phone down. I'm calm; my eyes are dry. We still have a lot to work out, but he's choosing me.

His final, simple text makes me smile. LOML—Love of my life. It's our thing.

I feel victorious when I lie down, like I've won the love contest, although I know none of this is real. Tomorrow will bring new drama. Chris is not good for me and we're not meant to be together. Yet, there's something I'm getting from him, from our relationship, that keeps me going back for more. I wonder if the day will come where I've had enough.

The feather pillow cradles my head and the sheets feel smooth against my skin. I curl onto my side and close my eyes, ready for sleep to come carry me into dreams of brighter tomorrows.

She is not worth it. Karen's words slice through my tranquil joy like a sharp knife through butter. My eyes open. *Fuck her. Who is she to say what I'm worth?*

I try to focus on my breathing like my therapist taught me: inhale for four counts, hold for six, out for four.

She is not worth it. Her voice is louder than mine.

An hour passes easily as I toss and turn. It's one in the morning, and then two. *She is not worth it*. The phrase keeps playing in my head; an earworm I'm powerless to stop.

It's nearly three when something jolts me awake. My eyes open to darkness. *She is not worth it*, I hear. But this time it's not Karen's voice I'm hearing; it's mine, and the phrase has changed. What I hear now is, *I am not worth it*. And with a sudden clarity I understand: it's always been my voice.

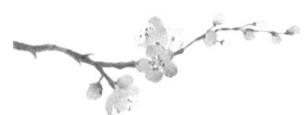

29

NOTHING TO LOSE

The one thing I do every day without fail, is pray. I don't know if that's why I've been spending less time in the weeds with Chris, or why my financial situation has changed for the better. But I can't argue that my life has improved since I started.

That doesn't mean it's been easy—far from it.

When I started praying a year ago, despite all my years of twelve-step program suggestions, I didn't know where to start. My experience with everything religious, which was what I believed prayer to be, was limited to what I'd learned as a child from Big Nana, my mother's mother. One night at her apartment, it was she who gave me my first lesson.

"Gail," she said in her deep, gruff voice before taking a long drag of her cigarette. I looked away from my card game laid out on her kitchen table. "I have to show you something."

Her expression was as serious as ever as she blew out the smoke.

She crushed her Winston in the glass ashtray and pushed back her chair. Then she rose from her seat at the head of the table with majesty, keeping her shoulders back as her leopard print turban stayed fixed on her head like a crown.

When she stood, I knew enough to follow her lead. I was on my feet by the time she lifted her large body fully out of the chair. This was all new territory, and I felt both anxious and excited about what she could have to share with me.

I followed her through the doorway behind me that led to her small bedroom. Its privacy curtain was pulled to the side, where it hung from a hook. She walked halfway into the room and stopped between the twin bed and tall dresser. Her husband, who was in the living room watching television, spent his nights there in his recliner.

Big Nana waited to speak until I was standing beside her. Her gaze was fixed on a statue that sat on top of the dresser.

"That's Mother Mary," she said without looking away from the dirty-white bust. "She's been crying. Can you see the tracks of her tears?"

I didn't need to look too closely to see that something was there. Below Mother Mary's right eye, a darkened line had been worn into the plaster like a dirt path into grass, running from the inside of her eye along her nose and stopping at the corner of her mouth.

Yes, I could see it as clearly as I could see Big Nana standing beside me, but I knew something wasn't right—I was ten, not stupid. Statues didn't cry. Still, I couldn't help but reach up to touch it and run my finger along the waterway. It was dry. I figured it was as good a time as any to ask about God, since nobody had ever told me anything about Him.

"Nana," I said, still looking at the statue, "where did God come from?"

She turned to me. "He just always was."

Well, that didn't make any sense. "He must've come from somewhere. Did he come from the clouds?"

"No," she said. "It's hard for us humans to understand because all we know is that there is a beginning and end. But God has always been."

I tried to grasp what she'd said, but thinking about it made my head hurt. The idea that anything didn't start somewhere was way more than I could comprehend. And although I hadn't known about Big Nana's mental health issues or her two years spent in the psychiatric hospital, I did know that she wasn't like other people. I left it at that and went back to my card game, while Big Nana went to get another beer.

Needless to say, Big Nana's crying statue didn't help provide me any direction. So when I started going to AA meetings at fifteen, less than five years after Big Nana's confusing lesson, I still had no real understanding of how prayer or spirituality was supposed to work. All I'd ever heard in AA was to "get on my knees," and I could say with absolute certainty, that I wasn't a get-on-your-knees-and-pray kind of girl.

In the beginning of my prayer life, I'd just lie in bed at night and think about what I would say out loud if I were talking to somebody else. Most nights, I'd fall asleep in the middle, but that was okay. I was doing it.

Mornings were different. Always in a rush, I'd multitask by praying in the shower or while driving to court, beginning the conversation with, "Good morning, God." Then I'd launch into whatever I thought necessary to have a good day. All I knew was I wanted to enjoy life and be a good person. "Help me stay away from drugs and cigarettes today. Help me to be kind, patient, and tolerant...."

Next thing I knew, I'd be thinking about the drunk driving case I had on that day or whether I'd paid my car insurance. Sometimes while driving, somebody would cut me off mid-prayer and I'd yell, "Hey, asshole, learn how to drive!" Even I knew this was not a great way to connect. It was so easy for me to lose track.

There had to be a better way, I was sure of that. Of course, I knew of many people who got on their knees. My ex-husband was a perfect example. Every morning and every night, he'd kneel next to the bed, bow his head, and talk to God. And he was staying clean. Then again, he was still so angry. So was that a better way?

And I wasn't a fan of the reasons people got on their knees. Some would say it was a way to humble themselves before God and to worship the Almighty. As far as I was concerned, I'd been humbled enough throughout my life—humiliated even—and whatever I was praying to hadn't given me any reason for reverence.

So I asked my therapist. Although Diana does her best to keep her religious ideas out of our sessions, I know she has strong feelings about God. So, in an afternoon session, I brought it up.

"I'm having a hard time with the whole prayer thing. I forget that I'm praying while I'm doing it."

"Do you get on your knees?"

"No, kneeling hurts me. I have bad knees." I didn't want to get into my real reasons.

"Have you ever seen the way Muslims pray?"

"No," I said, stifling a laugh. I certainly wasn't going to become a Muslim.

Diana surprised me when she got out of her chair, got down on her knees, and leaned forward until her forehead rested on her clasped hands on the floor in front of her.

"This is how they do it," she said, staying in position. "It's easy on the knees, and, more importantly, it keeps your heart above your head."

She looked absolutely ridiculous, and while what she'd said was logical, I would never do that. I was sure of it.

Later that same night, as I started my usual lying-in-bed prayer, the thought crossed my mind: What do I have to lose?

I slipped out of bed and onto the floor just as Diana had demonstrated. "I feel like a complete idiot," I said to the empty room, as though the admission would somehow ease my embarrassment. It didn't, but I kept going. I leaned forward and rested my head on my clasped hands. As soon as my forehead touched, I started to cry. It didn't make sense. I wasn't even sad. There were no memories of loss or heartache bubbling up to the surface.

Nothing.

But it didn't matter why. My body didn't care. Soon, I was sobbing. Tears drenched my hands and the rug below me. I held the position, not yet ready to break the connection that had evoked such raw emotion.

Several minutes passed before I could think again. I didn't know whether the emotional response had simply been the result of my willingness to try something different or my desire to change. That didn't matter either. I'd found a way to connect with what was inside of me. And I didn't have to define it, but I knew some things without question. It wasn't a guy in the sky. It didn't have a face or gender. It wasn't judgmental, and it didn't require worship.

"Thank you," I said, to nothing and no one in particular. "For all that I am and all that I have. Thank you for all the people who've touched my life. Thank you for all the experiences, even the painful ones." I thought of my mother, my father, and Chris. "Especially the painful ones. Thank you for keeping me alive long enough for me to recognize that I have value."

Since that day, every morning and every night, I get on the floor and let my forehead rest on my folded hands the way Diana showed me. While on the floor, I'm not distracted by other things, and I feel connected in a way I never have. There's no shame in that.

2012–2015

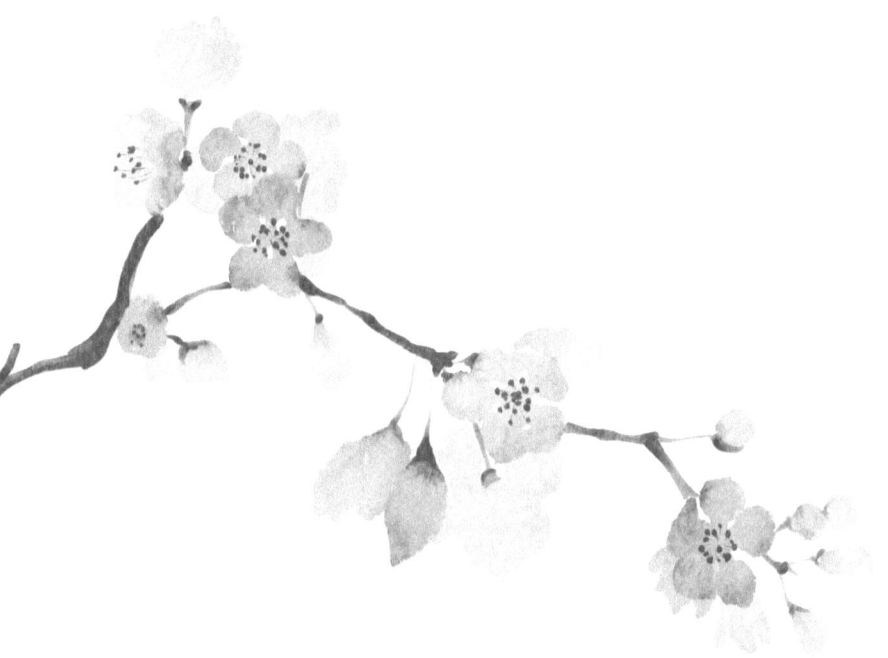

30

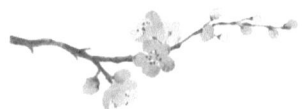

MOVE A MUSCLE

I did it! I jumped out of a plane. Now that it's over, and the stress and fear are gone, I'm left feeling invigorated. I'm ready for this next chapter in my life.

Move a muscle, change a thought. That's what I was thinking when I clicked "buy" on the skydiving Groupon. I'd been scrolling, looking for a discount on apple picking when the ad caught my eye. I needed to take action, and it had to be something big. I'd always thought so much about everything, but did so little to change. It was just the leap of faith I needed to take.

My friend Sandy was the first person I told. "I'm going skydiving."

"Are you crazy?"

"You know the answer to that question." I laughed.

"Do you want some company? I'm not crazy enough to jump out of a plane, but I'll go with you if you want." I was happy to have her come along for the ride.

In the days leading up to jump day, I wondered if I'd be able to go through with it when the time came. It wasn't like me to do something so reckless. I was just over forty, and until recently I didn't even like turbulence on a commercial airliner. Or takeoffs. Or landings, for that matter. In fact, the last time I did anything that felt as dangerous was when I was a passenger in my boyfriend's car while he drove up Mount Washington's winding road. I panicked and demanded he stop and let me out. I'd refused to get back in until he agreed to turn around and go back down.

Fear had also been my most prevalent emotion for the majority of my life. I had been afraid of absolutely everything—of being looked at and being seen. I was terrified of being remembered and also forgotten. I was afraid to be alone and of other people. I was afraid people would expect more from me than I could deliver or that I would be underestimated or overlooked. I was afraid to give too much or too little, to hold on or to let go. But what scared me most was that somebody would see how afraid I really was. So, I hid it well.

On the day of the jump, our small group watched a video, listened to a lecture, and suited up. We filed onto the small, seatless plane. As we taxied down the runway, I waited for the flight crew to close up the entrance, but it stayed open. I wondered how the plane could stay in the air with a big, gaping hole where a door should've been. It made me think of one of those movies where the airplane's cabin is peaceful, business-as-usual, until a bad guy detonates an explosive on the door, and everything not bolted down or belted in is sucked out the hole. Gratefully, that's not what happened.

I watched as the first guy lumbered to the door with the bulky parachute strapped to his back. He didn't have a partner. Then number two made the leap. I was next. The debilitating fear was gone, but I was afraid for sure.

As I stood in the opening, I thought about my kids and my sister. *I'll be fine*, I told myself. I also thought about Chris, and how he was probably with a new girlfriend, completely unaware I was about to jump out of a plane. Although I was sure he would feel terrible if I died, it would serve him right. I smiled at the petty thought.

"Are you ready?" my tandem partner yelled in my ear. He was crouched behind me, again checking the clips that bound us together.

"Ready as I'll ever be." That was the honest truth.

"Remember," he said, "it'll feel like you can't breathe, but you can. Right after we jump, pull your legs together and let them float out behind you. READY?"

But he didn't give me time to respond. A few seconds later, I was falling. It felt like I was suffocating as the man encircled my legs with his and pushed them behind us. I forgot all about my legs.

Within a minute, there was a cameraman floating in front of me, giving me the thumbs up.

"Give him a thumbs up," tandem guy said. So that's what I did.

A few seconds later, when the parachute opened, my body jerked upward. I inhaled sharply as the sudden pressure made the straps dig into my thighs with a pain that surprised the breath back into me.

Then, it was quiet. The only sound I could hear was the light wind on a perfectly warm September day. It felt as though the man strapped to my back and I were the only two people on the planet. For a moment, it didn't matter at all that Chris was probably sleeping in somebody else's bed.

Since making the jump, I'm wondering what new experience I'll have next. For so long, fear had me convinced that I didn't like change, so I didn't move too far away from the ordinary. I've heard people in meetings say, "There are two things I dislike most: when things change and when they stay the same." That's how I used to feel, like I was stuck either way. But I'm not, and I don't have to keep reliving the past. My days of fighting to survive are over.

I'm starting to see that change is a good thing.

I still don't have all the answers, but I'm finally asking the right questions— like whether I need a man to be happy. I'm starting to think I don't. And if I could fall through the sky at one hundred twenty miles per hour, maybe I can try spending some time with myself. It's definitely long overdue.

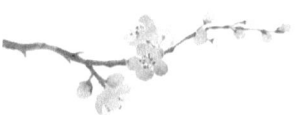

31

A NEW PATH

Warm water runs over my hands as I rinse the last mug. The dishes could've gone in the dishwasher, but I needed some busy work to occupy my mind, even if only for a few minutes. It's not working. No matter what I do, Chris won't get out of my head.

Regardless of how long we've been apart, I've yet to fully let him go. When he emailed last month to tell me he needed to change, I got excited. "I've been trying to get to new destinations while walking along the same old path," he'd said. I thought he was finally ready to stop getting high for good, but as it turns out, I was "the same old path." He had another new girlfriend a few weeks later.

It's still hard for me to imagine my life without Chris in it. I have this fantasy that true love will prevail against all odds and we'll find a way to be happy together. In times like these, when I'm most feeling his absence, I think only of the good times: us talking and laughing late into the night, camping with the kids, and spending weekends up north.

But those times were few and far between. The truth is that in the three years since we reconnected, we logged way more hours apart than together. Right from the beginning, Chris and I caused pain to all those who loved us. Our relationship was like a sinkhole, pulling in everybody around it when the ground gave way. After a while, most of my friends stopped coming close enough to risk falling in. And Ronnie still hasn't forgiven me. I'm not sure he ever will. Although during the last few months, we've been able to spend time in the same room without an argument breaking out.

I turn off the water and dry my hands. This obsessive thinking is enough to drive me mad.

Television is the only other thing I can think of for some quick relief. Mindless activity is the best way to avoid the things I'd rather not think about. Flipping through the channels—HGTV, Discovery, Lifetime—nothing catches my eye. Years ago, I might have made a call to a friend to gossip, complain, or to get lost in someone else's drama instead of sitting with my own pain. But I know none of those things will make me feel better. If only I could get out of here, go for a ride, but I can't. Serena is asleep upstairs. I should prepare my cases for tomorrow, but I can't focus right now.

After turning off the TV, I head back to the kitchen for a cup of tea. The ritual of making a cup usually soothes me. Normally, I love the sound of water pouring into my mug and how good the warmth feels when I wrap my hands around it. But not tonight. Nothing feels good to me tonight.

I need to *do* something. I'm a doer. At least, that's how I've always thought of myself. Now that I'm really thinking about it though, I'm wondering if I might be more of an avoider. My goal has always been to go over, under, or around a negative feeling instead of through it.

In every situation, I've asked, "What am I going to do?" Once, when I was in my early twenties and going through a breakup, I posed the question to a friend.

"You know, Gail," she replied, "sometimes the hardest thing to do is nothing." Her response startled me. Not once had it ever occurred to me to do nothing. It hadn't even been an option. I'm clearly still working on that.

As I sit at the kitchen table sipping my tea, looking as calm as can be on the outside, my head is spinning. I'm thinking about my mother and how similar we were. I wonder if I'm like her in this way too. She was also perpetually looking for relief. Walter was her Chris. Of course, she was also still getting high while she and Walter were together. Not that being drug free for over ten years has stopped me from using this obsession with Chris the same way I used fentanyl and Percocet. The way I'm still using the obsession. One way or the other, I'm avoiding. And using is using.

Maybe I'll just send him a text.

Without giving it another thought, I pick up my phone and open a new Chris text window. It's been a few days since we've had any contact.

Hey, I type. It doesn't deliver. He's blocked me again. Despite thinking I'm immune to the hurt from it, tears sting my eyes. As I feel the familiar weight of his rejection on my chest, I hear the words of my tandem skydiving partner:

"It'll feel like you can't breathe, but you can."

I can breathe.

But I have to do something. The hardest thing to do is nothing.

You could write. The thought pops into my head as though it's been waiting for its cue. Writing. Of course. Then I remember the book I started writing when I was twenty-four, after my boyfriend passed away. He was twenty-seven, way too young to die, and the loss of him left me devastated. He'd been gone for four months when I started to desperately type my story on an old word processor a friend had given me. Those first one hundred and fifty pages became the only thing standing between me and complete despair.

The thought of picking up where I left off excites me, like I'm about to go on a first date. But this feels more significant, unlike my usual distractions. Something about this feels important. Necessary even. The more I think about it, the more I'm convinced I should be writing.

I have to find that old manuscript. There's a version on my laptop that I transferred a few years ago from an old disk, but I need to feel the hard copy in my hands.

I begin my search in the basement, where I'm momentarily frozen by the sight of how many cardboard boxes are piled here. It's been quite a while since I've needed anything from these historical containers.

"One step at a time," I say out loud before getting to work. First, I set aside several large boxes belonging to Chris—old business documents, office supplies, remnants from when he had to close his shop. There's nothing personal in them, nothing I need to see, but I'm tempted. Having his things here feels like he's still part of my life somehow, and I really need to be free of him. I make a mental note to have him get them soon. The sooner the better.

Next, I move on to some other boxes, those containing what remains of my mother's worldly possessions. For a moment, I consider opening one of them for a quick visit with my memories of her, but I know I'll get lost in the past. Tonight is about moving forward. I'm on a mission.

When I open the first of my boxes, I'm met with a pile of journals and notebooks filled with my handwriting. I flip through them. While they contain an abundance of useful details about my life, the manuscript is not here. It's not in any of the basement boxes.

I move to the attic. Standing on the pull-down ladder, I open one of the two boxes placed precariously on the makeshift floor. And there it is. The manuscript is fastened neatly inside the report binder where I placed it seventeen years ago.

Laying the binder next to the box, I open to the first page. "11 AM and I could swear I heard a man call my name." Reading the words makes me smile. My obvious writing inexperience embarrasses me, but with so much of my story memorialized, I have a really good start here.

As sudden as a camera flash, I have a new sense of clarity. The pain I've known and my years of straddling addiction and recovery were all in preparation. My writing wasn't just meant to save my life back then; it was intended to be the beginning of something bigger. By sharing my experience, and showing people they don't have to live in shame, I can help them heal from their wounds. This is why my story has value.

My sister is the first person I call. I can hardly contain myself while I wait for her to answer. Gratefully, she picks up on the second ring.

"Chrissy," I say. "I'm going to write a book."

32

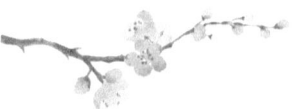

YOU ARE HERE

Walking through the aisles of the fabric store reminded me of how much I loved it there. It made me think of all the time I've wasted on nonsense like fear and drama. And when I looked at the fabrics, I saw possibility all around me. The idea of creating something from scratch excited me. It always has.

The last time I'd purchased fabric for a big project, it was for Alita's prom dress. I offered to make it, because that's what a good mother does. Several years clean by then, I was still trying to make up for the past, when I'd been high; present but absent at the same time.

After Alita chose the medieval design in deep purple velour and gold damask, I got to work. With the normalcy of having a husband and a home, I could spend my free time being creative. I worked night and day, until finally the dress, in all its glory, was complete.

"I love it!" she said, as I laced up the back. For the first time in her life, I felt like I was the mother she deserved. The dress was proof that when my mind wasn't consumed by chaos, I could be the mother I wanted to be.

That was over five years ago. In the time since, I'd filled every moment with marriage stress, the new house, and then relationship drama. There was no room left for creation. Now that I was on my own again, chaos-free, I was ready for another creative project.

And I had no intention of doing the same old thing. My plan was to try something new and bold.

First, I had to pick a pattern. As I thumbed through the catalogues, my eye was drawn to a short-sleeved dress; it was fitted at the top and flowing at the bottom, the kind that spread out wide during a spin. I didn't typically wear dresses, but my goal was to be different. I was, after all, trying on change.

Then, I chose my fabric. A bright yellow cotton captured my attention. It was perfect. I walked through the aisles with my shopping list: yellow thread, a zipper, lining, elastic, and a marking pencil. My eagerness to get started grew as I put each item in my basket with the cut material. Gathering these things made me feel like I had purpose.

When I got home, I laid everything out on the kitchen table, and a couple of hours later, I started putting it all together. That was just the beginning. There was still a lot of work to be done.

Over the next two weeks, I spent every spare moment on the project, just as I had with Alita's prom dress. This was how I wanted to use my time, creating instead of destroying. When I reached the end, when it was time to hand baste the hem by painstakingly pulling the thread through over a hundred times, I took it with me wherever I went. The dress was always draped over my lap and there was a sewing needle in my hand.

The process quieted my mind. When I was focused on measuring, cutting, and stitching, my thoughts stopped racing toward what happened the day before or what might happen tomorrow. I felt peaceful.

On the day my dress was finished, I slipped it on.

"Serena, can you come help me?" I yelled down the stairs.

"Oh, that's pretty," she said as she walked into the room. I turned so she could zip up the back.

"Why, thank you," I said, just like my mother would have.

When I spun around, the dress flared and rippled in a flash of yellow.

"I want a dress just like that," she said.

"We'll have to go to the store so you can pick a pattern and the fabric to make your own. I'll show you how." She was nine then, old enough to use a machine, and this was something I could give her.

She cheered with excitement.

Although I'd found some momentary peace while sewing, my mind still raced when I wasn't doing something. I'd been trying to meditate and sit with myself, but after a minute or less, I'd again start thinking about my childhood, or Chris, next week or a year from then. I needed to learn more about how to quiet my mind.

So I again asked my therapist for advice, since Diana had been so helpful when it came to prayer. I told her I wanted to have peace of mind, that I couldn't stop thinking, and that it got even worse when I was trying not to think.

She told me to focus on my breathing.

"There's no perfect way to meditate," she said. "It's all about being where you are."

Later that week, while in the nearby shopping mall, I passed by the map that showed all the store locations. There was a big red arrow that said, "YOU ARE HERE." I had one of those "light bulb" moments. I finally understood—that was what meditation was all about.

When I got home, I printed a large image of a red arrow I found on the internet, added the words I'd seen at the mall, and taped it to the wall in my home office. Then, I promised myself I'd keep learning.

AND SO CONTINUED my quest. Next came the books, YouTube videos, and conferences. I sought out spiritual teachers; one led to another and then another. That's how I ended up planning this trip to see Wayne Dyer.

A few days ago, the two Angelas, Serena, and I landed on the island of Maui. After a short ride from the airport, my sponsor, a friend from the program, and my little girl unpacked and settled into our shared ocean view room at the Westin.

Now, here I am on my last morning in Hawaii, feeling grateful that I didn't come with a man. Before now, all of my travel decisions had revolved around romance, and Maui, with its palm trees swaying in the breeze, waves crashing against the shore, and the sunset painting the sky pink and orange, is a perfect place for love. But I didn't come here for that—at least, not that kind. I came here to learn more about myself and to meet Wayne Dyer.

I first encountered Wayne at a conference in Atlanta a year ago, when I went with a friend during one of my lowest I-can't-live-without-Chris moments. While there, I heard him say, "You can't be lonely if you like the person you're alone with." It seemed like he was speaking directly to me and knew exactly how I felt. I'd been looking to spend time with somebody whose company I enjoyed more than my own. With such a low bar, all of my relationships had ended in heartache. How could they not?

Wayne began the first day of this Maui conference with meditation.

Because of the time change, I'd woken long before sunrise and practiced for fifteen minutes with a recording of Wayne reminding me to focus on my breathing. This was my second session of the day, so I already felt grounded. But I quickly learned that meditating in a room full of people has a different kind of power than meditating alone. Maybe it's the collective energy of a group that makes it easier to stay present.

Then, Wayne shared his teachings about how we can change our thoughts and our lives.

On the second day, at the end of the afternoon session, Mr. Dyer answered questions from the stage before ending for the day. I grabbed Serena's hand and rushed to the front along with several of the other hundred-or-so people in the room.

"Mr. Dyer, this is my daughter Serena," I said as loudly as I could without yelling. I knew he had a daughter named Serena too.

He looked at me, and then at her. He knelt down before us and addressed her as though she was the only other person in the room.

"Look at you," he said. "You are a gift." Serena smiled.

"I agree," I said.

"Are you having fun in Hawaii?" he asked her, all of his attention focused on her despite the crowd forming around the stage.

She nodded as I handed him the children's book we had purchased for him to sign. That moment was the kind I'd hoped for when planning the trip.

Yesterday, Serena and I had massages, a gift from Chris. "Use this for something to make you guys happy," he said as he pressed the hundred dollar bill into my hand at the airport. He's been trying to make things right between us. Maybe he's changed, but that's not as important as it used to be—I've changed. Although I'm not suddenly enlightened or completely free from repetitive thoughts, there are subtle differences for sure. I don't think the same way I did even a year ago, and being alone doesn't make me feel worthless.

Today, I'm the first one awake. As I sit on the veranda with my eyes closed, and soft music playing on my phone, a warm breeze carries the ocean air to me. My mother's words about building a foundation cross my mind. That's what I'm doing now—shoring up my foundation, making it strong enough to support me and my kids.

You are here. I smile.

33

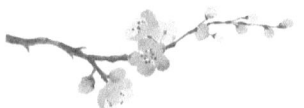

UNFAMILIAR TERRITORY

I hear the front door open and close, and my father moving around downstairs.

"Gail. Where you at?" he yells, his Texas twang so strong he could've been born and raised there instead of Gloucester, Massachusetts, where he lived until I was four or five.

"Shit," I whisper, letting out my breath. He didn't forget. I'd hoped I'd avoided the whole situation when I walked into the empty living room twenty minutes ago. It was 5:45, and our appointment was scheduled for six. Still, after scurrying up the stairs to the sanctity of my bedroom, I changed from my suit and started rehearsing what I'd say if he showed up. I've been sitting at my vanity doing just that. I don't know how to talk about my feelings, and the thought of telling him how sad and lonely I've felt my whole life because he wasn't around makes me feel nauseous.

"I'll be down in a couple of minutes," I yell back, but I stay seated, looking at my reflection in the mirror. All I can think about is how my father has never really been a part of my life. He moved down south when I was so young, I hardly remember him living nearby. The eighteen hundred miles between us would have been a long way if my father wanted me as his kid, but since he didn't, it made a relationship impossible. And his visits and calls were so rare, I was sure I didn't matter. How could I if my own father didn't want me?

Now, forty years later, there's a good chance I've been right all along, that I'm not important to him, and if I tell him how I really feel, he'll walk out of my life altogether. It's a silly fear, since he's never actually been in my life, but no amount of me trying to convince myself otherwise changes anything. I pretend like nothing's wrong. If he were to ask, I'd tell him I'm fine, despite the red-hot rage churning in my gut. But he doesn't ask. He's never asked, even though he's often the target of my sarcasm, a weapon that seeps out of me like gushing blood through a bandage. I still don't know how to communicate with him absent my shield of anger, and now that we have an appointment to talk, I don't think I can do it.

This wasn't even my idea. Not really. It all started when I stumbled across an ad for a year-long life coaching class at Boston University. I'd been thinking about changing careers for a few years, and coaching seemed like an easy transition from criminal defense work. I'd been feeling burnt out. I'd still be working with the public, and helping people, but unlike my position as an attorney, I wouldn't have to keep feeling like I was straddling two worlds—my professional one where I live as an attorney, and the poor, dark, addiction-riddled one that continues to live in me.

It's not that I desire complete secrecy. I'm okay with sharing some personal things, mainly about addiction, but the other stuff is way too shameful. I can't imagine what it would be like if those with whom I spend most of my days, court personnel, judges, and my colleagues, were to find out about the things I did with men for money when I was a kid, and that I have more in common with my clients than I do with them. I wish I didn't care so much about what they think, but I do.

Anyway, at class last night, we had to do a mock coaching appointment. I made the stupid mistake of agreeing to be the client. Luckily, there are only a dozen of us, all over forty, mostly women in the class.

As I completed my "Wheel of Life" pie chart, the instructor asked for a volunteer. Since my life success percentages were mostly low, I figured it couldn't hurt to get some feedback, especially since my relationship category was at a measly fifteen percent out of one hundred, and I was probably being generous with that. I thought it would be easy.

"Come on up," the instructor said. My "coach" was already sitting in her chair at the front of the room.

I took my seat across from her, fully prepared to play my part, already having decided I wouldn't give too much away. I handed coach Allison the chart and crossed my legs. For show, I was determined to appear as put-together as possible. Nothing new there.

She looked down at the chart and then at me.

"I see you gave your relationships a low score," she said.

"Yup. Story of my life," I said with a dry chuckle as I glanced around the room.

Straight-faced, Allison continued: "Who are your closest relationships right now?"

"My youngest daughter," I said. I kept my eyes on her as I answered, pretending the rest of the class wasn't judging me and my performance. Even though Chris is still the biggest reason for my low relationship score, I decided that was a situation better kept to myself. "And although I don't have a close relationship with my father, he's as close as he can get at the moment. He's here for a visit and he's staying with us." He'd shown up unannounced the week before.

"He's visiting?" she asked.

"Yes. He lives in Texas and doesn't come up this way very often."

"When was the last time you saw him?"

"Maybe five years ago. I'm not sure exactly. I'd have to think about it."

"Wow," she said, "that's a long time. It's got to be hard to be without your dad." The gentle way she spoke to me made my eyes fill with tears.

"Not really. He's never been a big part of my life. Hard to miss what you've never had."

"Does he know how you feel?" She looked at me so intently it felt like she could see my heart.

"I doubt it. I'm not sure he cares." As the words pushed the tears out, my hand instinctively moved over my mouth.

"Would you be willing to tell him how you feel? That might be a good place to start."

"I guess," I said, keeping my hand close to my face, a flimsy barrier between me and the audience. I would've said anything to get the session to end. Before I could get back to my seat, I had to have an "actionable goal."

"Will you schedule a time to meet with him?"

"Okay."

"How about committing to asking him to meet with you? Say, when you get home tonight?"

"I'll call him on the way home."

"And when would you like to have the conversation?" I didn't want to have the conversation at all, but I didn't say that.

"I'll see if we can do it tomorrow night when I get home, before he goes out to play pool."

"Perfect," Allison said, finally ending the exercise. The class applauded.

My relief to be back in my chair was short-lived. As my classmates took their turns, I thought about the conversation I'd agreed to have with my father. The more I thought about it, the more anxious I became.

Once on the highway, I dialed my father. When I got his voicemail, I hung up and thought about skipping it entirely; I could make up something to tell the class. They wouldn't know, and it wasn't like I was there for therapy. But in order to grow, I'd have to do things differently, which meant lying was out of the question.

My father was sitting on the couch watching television when I got home.

"Hey, Dad."

"Hey, sweetie," he said, in his jovial everything-is-a-okay-way.

"Is Serena asleep?"

"Well, she's been in her room for a couple of hours."

I took a deep breath and spoke quickly before I could lose my nerve. "I have to talk to you."

"What's going on?" he said as he reached for the remote and muted the television.

"I just need to tell you some things, but not right now. Let's talk tomorrow."

"Okay," he said, his eyebrows raised. It was odd to see him look concerned; it was an expression I'd never seen him wear.

"You're not going to play pool until later, right?"

"I'm fixin' to go out around six-thirty."

"How about six? Serena will be with Ronnie. I have work, and then I have some other things to do during the day." Half an hour would be plenty of time. I didn't want to leave any space for a potential awkward silence between us. I was also afraid he'd say something to hurt me more than he already had, and I'd have to sit there with him afterward.

"Okay," he said again. "Tomorrow at six."

Now tonight, if I could only think of a way to avoid going downstairs, I would. But these days, I'm trying to act with integrity, and a commitment is a commitment. And my father is downstairs waiting.

"You can do this," I say to the grown woman looking back at me—to the exact same deep blue eyes as my father's. But I'm talking to Little Gail, the part of me that has avoided this for years, and for whom this heart-to-heart is necessary. And I did promise myself while in Maui earlier this year that I'm willing to go through whatever pain I have to in order to change. I take a deep breath and head for the stairs.

My father looks up at me from the couch as I reach the bottom step. The television is off, and he's sitting as though he's been waiting for me. I really want to make a cup of tea, to ease into this thing, but even more than that, I want to get this over with.

I go directly to the loveseat on my father's right and sit with my feet flat on the floor in front of me. My father looks at me without speaking. This is brand-new territory for us both.

Looking down at my hands, I begin.

"When you moved to Texas and left me, it made me feel like I wasn't important enough for you to stay. It was like I didn't matter. My whole life, I thought I was unlovable." The tears burst out of me as I speak the last word.

Unlovable.

It's only recently I've been able to say it at all. My struggle with the word reminds me of the Fonz on *Happy Days*, and how he couldn't say sorry. He'd stutter every time. That's exactly how it feels to me.

The words gush out of me like a volcanic eruption that has been dormant for far too long. "I don't know why I wasn't enough for you to stay here. I was homeless, and a lot of people took advantage of the fact that I didn't have anybody looking out for me."

Other than what he's thinking, my only thought is whether it's always this quiet in my living room. I clear my throat just to make sure I can still hear.

When I turn to look at him, I'm surprised to see that his eyes are wet. In the forty-three years I've known this man, I've never seen him cry.

"Hell, Gail. I'm sorry. I had no idea you felt that way. I didn't leave you."

"You did leave me. Maybe things wouldn't have been different if you stayed, but my life was really hard."

He looks away, toward the window. "You were always important to me; I just didn't know how to be a father. I never learned how to take care of somebody else. All I really knew was to take care of myself."

I feel my shoulders relax as I exhale, noticing for the first time since sitting down that they were raised up to my ears like I'd been standing in the cold. I imagine this is what spring feels like after the winter thaw.

"I thought there was something wrong with me." I look down as the words bring a fresh stream of tears.

"There's nothing wrong with you. There never was."

When I look up again, although I know the man before me is my father, the eyes looking at me are filled with compassion, and I can't help but feel as though I'm looking at a stranger. Since I've never seen him express any real emotion, it occurs to me that I thought he lacked feelings. Now, I recognize the thinking as that of Little Gail.

"Thank you for saying that."

"I mean it," he says, looking me in the eye. It feels unfamiliar, and the uncomfortable feeling makes me look away. "I know I can't change anything, but I'm sorry."

His unexpected apology brings even more realizations.

My father is just a man. *How could I have not understood this before?* His apparent humanness feels like a revelation. *He didn't know how to do this life thing any better than I did.*

As we sit in silence, I close my eyes and scan my body for any trace of trapped feelings and things left unsaid, like an accident victim searching for injuries. There are none. The pain of untreated neglect has been excised, and my body feels nothing but relief. My father is sitting next to me, and I'm not bristling. With the resentment gone, what remains between us is love.

34

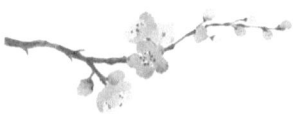

TRANSMISSION

I t's Tuesday night, and the small group of women who meet regularly at my apartment are spread out around the living room.

"Coffee?" Elaine asks before we get started.

"Yup. Next to the Keurig. There's tea in the cabinet too."

"I brought some cookies," Jess says. "They're in the kitchen."

A few of the women get up for snacks while the rest of us talk about our weeks. They're not only here for the meeting; some of them have become my best friends. In my nearly thirteen years clean, the circle of women in my life has grown, and this house meeting is one of the high points in my own recovery journey. Having these women here makes me feel more connected than when we meet in a church basement. That's what I want in my life: true connection. It's what I'd always wanted, but I didn't learn how to get it until this last year.

That's when I met Lisa at a Friday night meeting in New Hampshire. The blonde, petite woman sat at the front of the room telling her story without apology. She talked about the things she'd done, her four children, her multiple marriages. Her relationship history sounded like mine, but she seemed so respectable. It caught me by surprise. In all my years in recovery, it was the first time I wanted to be like another woman. Her insides seemed to match her outsides.

When the meeting ended, I made my way to Lisa through the crowd surrounding her. I felt the heat rising in my cheeks as I took a deep breath, steeling myself to ask for her help. I'd heard it said that asking for sponsorship was like asking somebody to be your Valentine, and that's exactly how it felt.

"Hi," I said. "I can relate to so much of your story. Would you be willing to sponsor me?"

"Of course," she said. It was that easy.

We started working together the following week. She showed me how to identify the ways I used people and things, and how to clear away guilt by making amends to the people I'd hurt. I learned about shame, my biggest problem, and I could see how it had been affecting every area of my life. Now I understood what my mother had meant all those years ago when she told me that "guilt is when you feel bad for something you've done, and shame is when you feel bad about who you are."

Soon, I was responding to situations in my life differently. No longer holding things in or lashing out, I started to feel better about myself and more connected to those around me. That gave me the strength to share openly about my shame. I stopped hiding the fact that I'd felt like I was worthless and unlovable. I said the words out loud, and became determined to share my whole story with the world. All of it. Even the parts about the men, the money, the dishonesty, and the fear.

Being vulnerable and sharing openly about my life allowed others to do the same.

Before long, I was showing other women how to make changes in their lives. I wanted to do for others what Lisa had done for me.

One afternoon, while working with a woman in my kitchen, I had an idea. We'd been talking about the need to identify the things that cause us problems; the things we hold onto despite the trouble they cause. I brought her over to my food pantry and opened the door.

"See how well-stocked it looks?" And it did. It was full. She nodded.

I removed a can of beans and looked for the sell-by date. When I found it, I read it out loud. It was outdated by six months. I reached for another. The next one was still good. I continued looking through, removing the few cans of beans, sauce, and boxes of pasta that had expired.

"Although it looks like I have less food, that's not really true since those items weren't good. I only removed the stuff that wasn't useful. Those things were only taking up space."

"That makes so much sense," she said.

"It's no different with what's on the inside. Once we identify those parts of ourselves that aren't useful, like anger, fear, and jealousy, we can clear them out and make space for creativity, compassion, and helping others. But first, we have to identify them."

As I spoke, I felt the truth of what I was saying. The transmission of knowledge and understanding had replaced a useless item I'd cleared from my inner pantry.

Tonight, we're reading from the *Big Book*. We're in the middle of a chapter when Serena comes downstairs.

I hold up my finger. "Hang on one second," I say to Stacy, who's mid-sentence.

"What's up, honey?"

Serena skips into the room. "Can I read?" she asks.

I look around for any sign of objection. There are none.

"Of course," I say, handing her my book.

She squeezes in beside me on the couch, and after I show her where we left off, she begins.

I listen with pride as she reads such a difficult text with few errors. She's grown so much in the five years since her father and I split up. We both have. As I look around the room, at the women with whom I share this space and my life, I know this is what I'm supposed to be doing, and this is why I'm here.

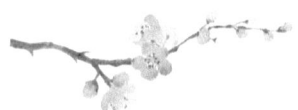

35

WHAT MATTERS MOST

For two weeks I agonized over a bottle of Advil. Since walking out of the big-box store without paying for it, I thought about the bottle constantly. Even though it was an accident, I felt like the thief I was in my younger years.

That night, while unloading the shopping cart into my Jeep, I found the bottle hiding behind my purse. At first, I wasn't sure if I'd paid for it. Cold and wet from the rain, I turned on the ignition and blasted the heat as I dug the store receipt out of my pocket.

The Advil wasn't on there. I hadn't paid for it. I looked toward the door, thirty feet away, and contemplated going back inside to pay for what now felt like contraband. "What to do," I said, more as a statement than a question. I knew it wasn't right to keep something I hadn't paid for, but the last thing I wanted to do was go back out into the rain. And given my money situation, I could've used a freebie.

For ten minutes, I sat contemplating. I knew I should brave the rain and go back into the store. As a woman in recovery from addiction, I'm supposed to "do the next right thing." But it was late, I was tired, and I really wanted to get out of those wet clothes. They wouldn't miss the bottle for one night, I reasoned. As I drove away, I told myself I'd go back the following day.

But I didn't. Not the next day, or the day after. And every day I put it off, I thought about it.

I mulled over something my therapist, Diana, had told me. She said that there are three parts that exist in all of us: the body, mind, and spirit, and that each part can be identified as the child (the body), the adult (our thinking), and the spirit (our conscience).

"Everything relates to these three parts," she'd said. "The child tells us when we need to be fed and nurtured or when we need to sleep. It acts on impulse, from muscle memory. And the adult, as the thinker and the judge, makes decisions. Then there's the spirit. It's the highest part of who we are, the voice from deep inside.

Picture a car. In a healthy person, the adult is driving, the higher self is in the passenger seat giving directions, and the kid is in the back. But with the addict, the child is driving, reacting to the world and the people in it. The adult is in the passenger seat trying to reason with the child and keep them in line. The higher self is in the back seat, trying to get a word in, but nobody's listening."

My car was clearly that of an addict. And Little Gail was driving.

I tried to drown out Diana's voice, but I kept coming back to honesty and my dysfunctional relationship with money. My finances were still a mess. I thought about the trips to Manhattan and Vancouver I couldn't afford but took anyway, and about my recent brush with having my Jeep repossessed.

Six months before walking out with the Advil, I'd gotten a letter from my credit union saying they'd be sending someone to collect either my Jeep or the seven hundred and sixty-five dollars I owed them.

As promised, a man knocked on my door late that Friday afternoon. I invited him in and handed him an envelope full of cash. He counted it quickly but carefully.

"This isn't enough," he said.

"What do you mean? That's what they said I had to pay to get caught up."

"Yes, that's what would have caught you up before the credit union recalled the loan. The only way for you to keep the car is to pay the loan in full."

"Well, how much is that?" I asked, my voice shaky.

"Seven thousand six hundred forty-two dollars."

My legs felt so weak I feared they'd give out.

"But I don't have that kind of money. I'm a single mother, and if I can't drive there's no way I'll be able to work."

"Listen," he said, "I don't want to make your life any harder than it is. I'll tell the bank that the vehicle wasn't here. That'll buy you a few days. Try going to the higher-ups and see if you can work something out."

After he left, I knew I had to show the lender I was serious about getting my life together. That's when I thought about the book I'd been working on. I printed my manuscript and slid the thick stack into a white envelope. The following Monday, I went to the credit union's main office. After explaining my situation and showing him the manuscript as proof of my determination to become financially stable, the head loan officer agreed to restructure the loan. I haven't been late on a car payment since.

A couple of months after that, the IRS came after me for back taxes: close to forty grand. Self-employment brought a whole new set of requirements and obligations I didn't know how to navigate. Another result of my upbringing, I'm sure, but that's no excuse. I am, after all, an adult. I was able to work out a payment plan that I'm still trying to keep up with in addition to my regular bills and student loans.

But that's not why I hadn't been back to the store. Part of me had hoped I'd just forget about it. I figured wrong. There are all kinds of ways to steal, and even though I hadn't taken the bottle on purpose, keeping it would've been intentional. And I knew the longer I waited to make the situation right, the more ridiculous I'd feel doing it.

That's why I'm here today.

When I walked into the store, I went directly to the medicine aisle and got the same bottle I'd walked out with, and brought it to customer service.

"I was here a few weeks ago and accidentally walked out with one of these," I said. "I want to pay for it, and I figured it would be easier if I brought you one so you'd know how much it is."

"What?" the clerk asked, her forehead crinkling. "You're not buying this?"

"No, I already have one at home."

"But you want to pay for it?"

"Yes," I said, smiling.

"Why would you bother paying for it now?"

"It's the right thing to do."

Sitting here in the quiet of my Jeep, I feel lighter than when I arrived. I wasted so much time and energy these last couple of weeks, when I could've just addressed the situation right away. Of course, it was never about the Advil.

The bottle was just a symbol for all the things I do and the ways I behave that take my attention away from what's important.

I'm finally starting to get it. Without those thoughts taking up space in my head, I can focus my attention on what matters most: my family, work, and writing. Freedom is what I get from keeping my pantry clean.

36

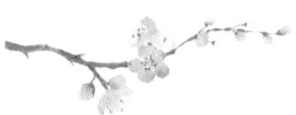

CHOICES

Cancer. That's what the doctor said. "From what I can see, this looks like it could be a rare form of cancer."

There had to be a mix-up. I'm the one with the rash, I wanted to say. I stayed quiet, sure she'd figure it out. But I couldn't take the silence and the expectant way she was looking at me.

"Cancer?" I finally asked.

"I can't say for sure, and I don't want to alarm you, but if I'm right, it's quite serious. This isn't my area of expertise, but what I do know is that this is how inflammatory breast cancer presents. I'm going to schedule some tests. You'll need a mammogram, ultrasound, and biopsy right away; within the next few days. This kind of cancer is very aggressive. Do not put this off."

I watched her mouth move while she spoke, and despite us being the only two people in the room, it felt like she was talking to somebody else. As hard as I tried to follow her words, I couldn't stop thinking about how I'd been right all along—I was going to die at forty-five like my mother.

And what about Serena? She needed me. No ten-year-old should have to grow up without their mother, and I'd always promised I'd be there for her the way my mother hadn't been there for me.

"Do you have any questions?"

She was definitely talking to me.

"I can't think of anything." That was the truth.

"Okay. You can get dressed and stop at the referral desk on your way out."

When I looked in her eyes, I could see the sadness in them. The doctor put her hand on mine before she spoke again. "I'm sorry to have to give you this news."

THAT WAS IN May of last year. Eight months later, I started radiation, the third and final leg of treatment. The schedule was set—radiation five days a week for six weeks.

Each weekday during the last five weeks, a technician started my music playlist while another got me into position. Then, for twenty minutes, while my arm was raised above my head, the machine worked its magic.

Three days ago, near the end of my fifth week of radiation treatment, I was in tears as I begged the doctor to stop the treatment. I rarely complained about the pain, but the high-test burn cream, the kind they give third-degree burn patients, had stopped giving me relief.

"We can't stop," Dr. Frank, the radiation oncologist, said. "We've found that the rate of success is less if we don't complete the whole six weeks. But I will give you a break. I'll let you take a long weekend, four days instead of two. We'll get back to it on Tuesday. I'll also write you a prescription for the pain," he said, smiling sympathetically. "Come out after you get dressed."

I found Dr. Frank waiting for me in the hallway.

"Here's your prescription," he said as he handed me a small square of paper. "I wrote it for eight. Don't take them all at once," he chuckled. If he only knew that thirteen years before, I would've taken five of them right away. The entire prescription would've been gone by mid-day, and I'd be calling for more. I took the script, folded it in half, and put it in my purse.

"I'll try not to," I joked. He didn't know anything about my sordid addiction history. And he didn't need to know. As an adult, it was my problem, not his.

A few minutes later, I was back in the sanctity of my car, one step closer to being home where I didn't have to act like I was okay.

After starting my Jeep, I pulled out the prescription. Doing this felt like part of an old ritual. "Holy shit!" I said aloud when I realized I'd misheard Dr. Frank—he said eighty, not eight. That's why he made the joke.

As I studied the prescription, I thought about my mother. Although she'd stopped using heroin a couple of years before she died, she relapsed a few months before her last trip to the hospital. She wasn't trying to stay clean anymore. Her battle with addiction was over. She was tired, lonely, and in pain, she'd said. I knew exactly how she felt, and relief was in my hands.

And my pain was legitimate. The mastectomy had been brutal. They'd removed not just my breast but all the lymph nodes under my arm as well. Now the radiation had burned my chest so badly that the skin was peeling away in sheets. Even wearing a bra was agony, but I couldn't leave the house without the prosthetic. Every movement sent fire through my chest.

It was the second time I needed painkillers since getting clean. I had to take some after the mastectomy, but once the pain subsided, I switched to ibuprofen. But back in November, during the surgery, I wasn't living alone. Now, I didn't have any choice but to handle the pills on my own.

The first stop I made was the pharmacy. The pharmacist's eyes widened when I handed him the prescription. With my buzz-cut, and my eyebrows only just starting to grow back, I was obviously a cancer patient. He knew I needed them.

"Can I just get some of the pills, and if I need more, come back and get them?" I asked. I knew I wouldn't need them all.

"No," he said. "Whatever you don't take, you lose."

For a moment, I considered having him give me just twenty or thirty, but it seemed blasphemous to give them up. And what if I did need them? The pain was excruciating, and I had no idea how long it would last.

"Just fill the whole thing then," I said with a wave of my hand.

FINALLY AT HOME with my massive bottle of pills, I headed straight for the kitchen to wash down a Percocet. I was desperate for the relief that would soon come.

I added the bottle to the rest of my cancer medications and paraphernalia in the hall closet and lay on my bed to wait. In the meantime, I couldn't help but think about all the ways I was failing Serena.

She needed me. As a child of divorce, living with me as her primary caretaker, she'd had a hard enough time before cancer. I was certain that at ten, my little girl must've wondered what would happen to her if I didn't survive. And I didn't know what to tell her. I wasn't afraid to die, but I was terrified to leave Serena the way my mother had left me. If not for myself, I had to be okay for her.

Over the last couple of days, since starting the Percocet, I've been spending most of my time at home alone with the pills. With my caseload light and my income supplemented by donations and fundraisers, my main job is to recover. Gratefully, Serena has been with her dad and her friends, which gives me the space to heal. But the pills are always on my mind.

No matter what I'm doing, whether it's watching TV, taking a shower, or washing the dishes, they creep into my thoughts. It's as if there's an energy between us, and I wonder if they sense me the way I sense them.

The prescription allows for two pills every four hours, but I haven't taken nearly that many. Unlike in the past, I don't even like the way they make me feel. Before, a few pills gave me energy—I could clean my entire apartment in a few hours. Now they leave me feeling like I'm underwater, sluggish and foggy, with a stomachache and constipation. I can see why non-addicts would stop taking them. But even that doesn't stop me from wanting the drugs.

Several times a day, when I walk by the closet, I open it to make sure the bottle is still there. Every so often, I take it out, feel its weight in my hand, and count what remains. As of this moment, end of day two, there are seventy-four pills left. Of course I already knew that. In less than three days, they've again become the focus of my life.

That's how I know it's time for them to go.

My first thought is that I should sell the pills. Just because I don't want to get high anymore doesn't mean there aren't plenty of people who'd love to get their hands on Percocet. Their street value is about the same as when I was actively using them. I can get ten dollars each, no problem. That would mean over seven hundred dollars in my pocket.

"That's old thinking," I hear myself say. I can't side with addiction and put drugs in somebody else's hands for any amount of money. It's taken so much from me and the people I love. If I'm going to stay clean, I can't live dirty.

I'll drop the bottle off at the pharmacy tomorrow, I decide, as I wash down another pill.

My FULL BLADDER jars me awake at three o'clock in the morning. Groggy as I make my way to the bathroom, I swear I hear the whisper of my name as I pass the closet and the Percocet. I'm suddenly wide awake. Maybe I should take one, I think, since I'm getting rid of them tomorrow. But I'm not in pain, at least not enough to warrant a painkiller.

Still, I check on them. In the closet, the bottle sits exactly where I left it, looking innocent enough. I pop off the cap so I can see the chunky white pills. I'm torn. I feel so much for them, both desire and anger. They saved me at a time when, without their relief, I would've taken my life. But then they became everything to me. I couldn't begin the day without them, and did whatever I had to do to satisfy my need for them. It was beyond my control. They were my salvation and my enemy.

But deep down, I know they're part of the problem, not the solution. And I alone have to decide whether to embrace them or let them go. There's nobody to stop me.

Moving quickly before the craving can take hold, I step into the bathroom, lift the lid, empty the bottle into the toilet, and flush.

For today, at least, I choose to stay clean *and* live clean.

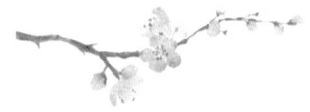

ACKNOWLEDGMENTS

There are several people who deserve thanks for helping bring this book into the world. If I've left anyone out, please forgive the oversight—memory has its limits. Also, independent publishing isn't the solo act it appears to be. This book exists because of a collaboration, and I'm grateful to all who contributed.

To my kids: Artemis, Jack, and Serena, who never once complained when I chose to share our story with the world, thank you for your trust and your courage.

Thank you to my sister Chrissy and my brother-in-law Michael Lattanzi, for not only being part of my story, but the best beta-readers as well. Your attention to detail and feedback have been essential.

Deb Goldstein, my friend and writing coach: you pushed me when I needed pushing, listened when I needed to talk it through, and helped me figure out what this story was really about.

My friends, Jules Griffiths, Jenny Cutler, Sierra McGregor, Kristen Belleville, and Michelle Doucette, thank you for reading and for believing in this book and in me.

And to Lisa Hart-Martin, who helped me learn how to stop "living dirty." This book wouldn't exist without you.

For those who found themselves part of my story without choosing to be, I know that wasn't easy, and I'm sorry for any pain I caused. Your presence in these pages comes with gratitude for what you taught me, even when the lessons were hard for both of us.

Finally, as always, thank you Kenny Francis for cooking me meals and for helping me get this book out into the world. I'm incredibly grateful to have you in my life.

To everyone who read *The Fruit You'll Never See* and waited for me to finally finish this one, your patience didn't go unnoticed. Thank you. I'm already at work on the next one.

gailnastasia.com

www.ingramcontent.com/pod-product-compliance
Lightning Source LLC
Chambersburg PA
CBHW021145130626
46554CB00005B/1679